BETWEEN

There is a Difference
Living the Between of Mental Health

MICK HUMBERT

authorHOUSE·

AuthorHouse™
1663 Liberty Drive
Bloomington, IN 47403
www.authorhouse.com
Phone: 833-262-8899

Published by AuthorHouse 08/17/2022

ISBN: 978-1-6655-6799-2 (sc)
ISBN: 978-1-6655-6800-5 (hc)
ISBN: 978-1-6655-6798-5 (e)

Library of Congress Control Number: 2022914966

Print information available on the last page.

All Bible references are from the The Holy Bible, Modern English Version. Copyright © 2014 by Military Bible Association. Published and distributed by Charisma House.

This book is printed on acid-free paper.

Dedication

To all those who live with, and who support those who live with,
the between of Mental Health

Gratitude
For the editing skills of John Becker and Melanie Howard

Citations
All Bible references are from the World English Bible translation
Permission received from other contributing authors

CONTENTS

Introduction...ix

THE CRISIS

eviL - Live 1
Listless - Lifeless 3
Giving Up - Surrender.. 5
Time's up - Time Out.. 7
Death Sentence - Life Long... 9

THE TRIP

Gravel - Smooth Asphalt 13
Hide - Run.. 15
Passenger - Driver 17
Sprint - Marathon 19

THE LOVED ONES

Foe - Friend... 23
Sympathy - Empathy... 25
Knowledge - Knowing 26
Absence - Presence... 28

THE MODALITIES

Being a Pill - Taking a Pill.. 33
Dead Food - Live Food 35
Mindless - Mindful 37
Wiped Out - Exercise 39
Answers - Avenues 40

REALIZATION

Expertise - Experience 43
Desperation - Perspiration 44
Hopeless – Hope 45
Why - Wisdom 46

INTRODUCTION

A poem, and its ongoing impact on millions of people, produced a "click" in my head for what you are about to read. That poem is "The Dash" by Linda Ellis, written one afternoon in 1996. Even beyond its profound message and words, the life observations that inspired this poem prompted an "ah-hah" moment and a nod of my head.

So, I write, not with any vision of some far-reaching impact, but from my observations born of over 30 years of lived experience with a Mental Illness. I wrote a book called *Bicycles Built for the Blues* around the time of my first in-patient treatment in 2015-16. Over the next three years, and four in-patient visits culminating in eleven Electroshock Therapy sessions, I wrote a book with other contributing writers who were affected by my Mental Illness, called *One Flight into the Cuckoo's Nest*. Now six years removed from that initial Psych Ward stay, I consider what I have felt and experienced on the continuum between Mental Illness and Mental Health. Following another relapse in early 2022, I received another 10 Electroshock Therapy sessions. All three writings are contained in this book, and they constitute my attempt at describing a life lived in "the between" of Mental Health.

If I may be so bold, like "the dash," there is "a between" that I observe, feel, and cry with. In hindsight, this has made all the difference in still being alive and vertical after over 30 years with a Mental Illness. This is not hyperbole for me. Beyond staying married for almost 40 years and raising two daughters to move forward in their own lives, I count being alive and vertical as my greatest accomplishment in life. I have found a way or ways to continue to live, even when the temptation to end the seemingly endless suffering has been all too real.

In other writings, I have identified this accomplishment as being a "warrior," a description borrowed from a woman who described herself as such in a treatment program that I was also a participant in. Warriors with a Mental Illness win some and lose some of the daily battles, but without a doubt there seems to be a daily conflict or friction of varying degrees between Mental Health and Mental Illness. I think this is true for everyone, it's just that those who manage a Mental Illness are more acutely aware of it. For me, being a warrior with a Mental Illness is certainly not a badge of honor, but neither am I guilt-ridden or ashamed of having a Mental Illness, as I once was.

Thankfully, the research and knowledge within the Mental Health profession is ever- expanding, but it is only one perspective. What is missing is the viewpoint and wisdom of those who personally manage a Mental Illness. More and more individuals are coming forward with their stories, but although great wisdom and insight can be gleaned from them, it is only a whisper so far. So, I add one more whisper in this book; a view after 30+ years and counting of dealing with a Mental Illness while in a present state of relative Mental Health and remission of my illness. The new material in this book is broken down into a number of categories with topics in each. I have no doubt that, depending on who you are and the perspective that you bring with regards to Mental Health, some categories will be more meaningful than others. I am not a Mental Health professional, nor do I claim to be one. But that does not minimize the voice and input I claim with regard to my own Mental Illness, and whatever assistance or impact my "sacred story", as I call it, may have on others.

This book is laid out in three segments: "Between", written from a state of remission that was interrupted by a third major relapse in health since 2022; "One Flight Into The Cuckoo's Nest", written in 2020, a year into remission after a three-year period of relapse; and "Bicycle Built For The Blues", written in the midst of the initial major relapse in early 2016.

How can one be contemplating suicide, but also contemplate and fulfill a number of advanced educational degrees? Some might say there is nothing intelligent about suicide. How can one not have the energy or will to continue with life, but also push oneself to bicycle over a thousand miles multiple times? Some might say both spectrums are "crazy." How can one be locked up with their shoelaces and belt removed for safety, but also assist others in unlocking importance in life as a social worker and Chaplain? Some might say a social worker or Chaplain has no right to assist others when they cannot even assist themselves. One premise behind this book is that similar extremes can and do exist, and more commonly in our human condition than one might think. Why? Because humanity, indeed the brain, is natural, mysterious at times, and very complex.

Between you and I, welcome to the "between" of Mental Health and Mental Illness as I presently see and experience it. My only suggestion in reading the following is to not think of the juxtaposed terms as good vs bad. Rather, be open to the notion that within them lies the spectrum and reality within which a person journeys in life, especially a person who lives with and manages a Mental Illness.

THE CRISIS

MICK HUMBERT

Healing is only partly about the wounds,
for the scars often remain

---

eviL - Live

Breathing, check. Heart pumping, yep. Mind working - sort of. Living well - definitely not. An out of body, certainly out of one's mind experience - absolutely. Explaining my Mental Illness to someone during a significant relapse has been and always will be difficult. What I do know is that I am not my normal self. In my case, it starts with anxiety and ends in panic and/or depression within a very short period of time - a matter of days to a week or two. Feeling the weight of my crisis, my stomach can't handle the situation, and I lose weight fast. There is a singular focus - panic and obsession, if you will- which I can just as easily describe as evil. Mental Illness is a natural process, but make no mistake: there is little redeeming about it in times of significant relapse. Put simply, the further away one gets from the will to live, the more evil life becomes.

Some similarities with Alzheimer's and Dementia, make some sense to me. I worked as a Chaplain in a Senior Living facility, which included Memory Care units. Loved ones, especially spouses, often describe their family member or spouse as almost unrecognizable in the emotional sense - present physically but not mentally and emotionally. Using spiritual language, I might say that there is a disconnect between the body and soul. It has been similar for me during a Mental Illness relapse. I am physically present and look normal, but I am not really there at all, or I must strain mightily to simply be present emotionally and mentally.

The common thread I have garnered from my own experience, and most certainly from listening to others who suffer from a Mental Illness, is that one is not themself. They have lost touch with life and living. Whether a slow erosion, or a quick plummet, as is my case, the capacity to live has been turned towards its opposite, or so it seems. "Live" now feels backwards, something we might render as "eviL".

Whether healthy or at significant dis-ease, we all function within the spectrum from truly alive to something not so, something eviL. There is a difference, a very significant one, perhaps affecting the core of one's purpose and being.

Listless - Lifeless

It might seem that both of these terms are similar, and similarly tragic, but I view them differently. When things seem lifeless, there is an absence of that which normally engages the mind, body, and soul under healthier circumstances. These things, whether they are individuals, items, or situations, are no longer engaged in. But nonetheless, they continue on without us. It may seem unfair and cruel; that life continues on no matter what is personally going wrong. However, in that continuance of life lies hope, memories of times when you were a full participant in life. No matter how dire any situation was for me, that hope was the thread - sometimes the only thread - that I hung onto when I was in the midst of a Mental Health crisis. Potentially, there could be a return from the pain and despair that I was experiencing during a Mental Health relapse. What I was going through was not the norm; something else did indeed exist.

For me the category of being, which I label here as listless, is much more dangerous and life threatening. The body, mind, and/or spirit is severely threatened. The will to move, the will to think, and the will to hope have gone limp. Thoughts as they are, plentiful to the point of obsession, solely focus on the situation at hand. There is a belief, from the core of one's being, that there is no way forward but staying in the present is not an option either. At first a mere whisper, it grows into an inner conversation around the viability of one's life. Pushing it away, or welcoming distractions, can and does delay the seeming inevitable. But listlessness has now become the predominant state of being.

I believe that everyone, and I mean everyone, has a limit of the physical, mental, and/or spiritual pain that they can endure. Once that endurance is exhausted, no matter how supportive one's environment and support systems are, listlessness can enter and demoralize one's desire to continue. Continue with relationships? — "The sounds in my head are deafening, much less having to listen to others." Continue with hobbies? — "But that would take energy." Go for a walk? — "I'd rather curl up in a corner or just pull the sheets up over my head." Just eat something? — "I feel nauseated and my stomach aches." What about the happier times and accomplishments of the past? — "They don't matter." At least continue breathing? — "Thankfully it is an involuntary impulse, because I feel I am suffocating in my thoughts of gloom and doom." The listless list can seem endless.

Therefore, I believe there is a difference between these two terms. Parts of our life — relationships, family or work for instance can be lifeless, yet our thread of hope remains. By contrast, when the fight is waged within the core of one's being, we have entered a very dark place, in fact, the darkest place I have encountered. In my relative Mental Health following remission, I am motivated to avoid visiting that darkest of dark places again. Why? Fear for sure, but also a desire to experience life again, normalcy of relationships and events, even if they can seem lifeless at times.

> Who you surrender to makes a difference. Giving
> in and abdication is not the same as giving up.

Giving Up - Surrender

Giving up means to me a personal and private abdication, saying, "No more." It is full and complete withdrawal from the struggle, even losing the will to live. It has much in common with being listless. Surrender, on the other hand, means to me the willingness to give in to the reality of my Mental Illness, and to engage others so that they may assist and potentially save me when I am in no condition to do that for myself. I surrender myself into the care of others.

This state of abdication that is "giving up" can take a number of forms, perhaps to varying degrees, in a variety of situations. I was once taking care of my two-year-old daughter, when all at once I sat up against a wall and wept. Many a night I got up at night so as not to wake my wife, and cried in another room. For all too many people, giving up can lead to a wish to pull the trigger, or in my case thoughts of driving my car at high speed into a barrier. If suicide is successful, there may be a simple note to others that says, "I am sorry, it won today." But for way too many, there is not even a note, no conversation with anyone about a crisis of health, just one final lonely decision.

A couple years ago, I was a guest presenter via Zoom on suicide prevention for the employees of a Minnesota state department. In the beginning, the moderator asked everyone for a single word that comes to mind when hearing the word "suicide". One participant said, "Apathy." Initially I was stunned by the suggestion, since my personal experience was the opposite. But I accepted that apathy might make sense to an outsider to Mental Illness. In not caring any longer, in giving up and ending one's life, apathy could be viewed as an appropriate description. But leading up to that moment of crisis - at least in my experience, and those of others I have listened to in Mental Health programs; - it is anything but apathetic.

Yes, everyone has their limits. A Mental Illness, if strong and prolonged enough, can wear you out physically, mentally, and emotionally. Our mind, the precise organ that is needed to whisper, "Hang on," is also the organ that is in dis-ease and yells back, "But why?" I am short on advice, but I do know that a fateful decision lies ahead for a person in such a critical state. In a moment or moments of brief clarity, does one decide to surrender into the care of others or not? As a person fortunate enough to have done so a number of times and come out the other side into remission, all I can say is that it can work. If you can no longer help yourself, your surrender will allow others to do so on your behalf.

Why are we so willing to give others time to heal, but we are reluctant to allow ourselves the same grace?

Time's up - Time Out

How much time is your Mental Health worth? Even more critically, how much time is your life worth? The surrender to a Mental Illness has a time factor to it; one must allow time for oneself to be ill. In other illnesses, such as cancer, stroke, or heart attack, the need to take time to be ill and to recover is well accepted. Allowing others whatever time is necessary, even from a job, is typically an empathetic response to such illnesses. It is the accepted course of action from loved ones, the ill person, and a vast majority of employers as well. Unfortunately, the need to deal with a Mental Illness is not nearly so empathetically appreciated. In another part of this book, I will address the role of others, but here I will address the factor of time for anyone suffering with a Mental Illness.

When in a Mental Health crisis, there is little time for the past or the future, because the illness takes up all of one's time - in thought, emotions, and sense of physical well-being. In fact, the crisis might be so severe that one could feel that time is running out. In this place of desperation, suicide might seem like a real option. Hence the question: how much time is your health and life worth? Will a person take time off work? Will they swallow their pride soon enough to put themselves in the care of others? Will they dare try something, anything, if suicide becomes a real option?

Of course, the answer to those questions from a rational state of mind would be, yes. But as stated previously, that is exactly the difficulty of a Mental Illness: the mind needed for such rational thought is now dis-eased to the point that rational thought might not be likely. It is a wicked conundrum, in fact, it is eviL. In such an environment, one might consider the image of a child in a mischievous moment, who needs a "time out". A wiser and older mentor, typically a parent, takes charge of the child to give them time to cool off and think of a better way forward. Something, anything, needs to change, because the present bout of misbehavior is intolerable. To another room the child goes, with a parent checking in frequently to see if and how the situation has changed.

While I am now perfectly fine with applying that image to myself, years ago I was too proud to be that humble or self-aware. When my mind has a fit and is misbehaving badly, I need a very serious and deliberate time out. Just before I wrote this chapter in January 2022, I had a partial relapse of my Mental Illness. With an imminent vacation to a southern climate with my entire family, the question arose whether I should go and battle through the symptoms in California or connect with my psychiatrist, in case the symptoms got severe enough to warrant ECT treatment. My wife and I decided to go on the vacation, a "time out" of sorts, while connecting with a specialist in case I would need to fly back home for ECT treatment. This was not the family vacation I had envisioned. But the sun, warmth, plenty of walking, meditation/ prayer to even out the significant anxiety symptoms, and a supportive spouse helped settle the symptoms. The cloud of my Mental Illness, that had been building into a severe storm, abated, and the skies cleared for another month. Time outs can take a variety of forms, but some sort of significant time out is necessary in such situations. I believe the common thread through them all is that enough time should be allowed to be ill and to recover while in the personal care of loved ones and/or professionals. Yes, - swallow your pride and take a time out.

Death Sentence - Life Long

This topic of a Mental Health crisis has been intense, and even deadly serious. For some, across all walks of life, choosing to end one's life becomes an option. Statistically, suicide is around the 10th leading cause of death in the United States, and the 15th throughout the world. Once, when I was in inpatient treatment, I became aware of another chilling statistic: one of every ten persons admitted to an inpatient facility in the United States for Mental Health will commit suicide. Yes, Mental Illness is a deadly serious topic.

In addition, this is an illness for life. Yes, individuals can have long periods of remission, but relapsing into symptoms of the illness, even a crisis is always possible. Typically, remission of a Mental Illness takes incredibly hard work - physically, emotionally, and spiritually. To get back to living, I believe that a person with a Mental Illness must come to grips with it being a lifelong reality. A person who does not have to like it, but they must own reality. Only they can begin the process of finding, developing, and honing some combination of coping skills, professional help, and medication assistance if needed. It has taken me over 30 years to develop a healthy strategy to manage my Mental Illness, and the process will never be finished. More than once, I mistakenly thought that Mental Illness was in my past, but relapses have taught me that I can never take anything for granted.

It is a cruel reality to live between the boundaries of a death sentence and a life-long illness with potentially deadly consequences, but the life of the dis-eased mind is cruel at times. To be fair, there is cruelty involving the mind in many other things as well. I will mention a couple, because considering similarities with other situations or conditions seems to help others more readily grasp the reality of Mental Illness when I describe my experience. The potential for having a relapse in Mental Health has some similarities with a person who has cancer in remission but who waits upon each regular blood test or scan to see if the cancer has come back. Since I suffer from Seasonal Affective Disorder, my regular "test" is winter; only during northern American winter months have I had severe symptoms and/or a relapse.

With a cycle of remission and relapse, whether regular or irregular, comes the deep mental scar tissue of the pain and suffering experience. In one of the outpatient treatment programs I was in, the visual analogy used is the deep worn path of Mental Illness with tall grass on each side. It triggers the, "Oh nooo, is it coming back again?" I also notice similarities to descriptions of the effects of PTSD: deep emotional and mental scars, triggers, and the well- worn path of symptoms.

I cannot change the reality that I have two life-long illnesses or conditions, probably interconnected: chronic back pain and a Mental Illness. It is one of my main journeys in life that I have embraced and made adaptations for. So, to that trip, that journey with a Mental Illness, I now turn.

THE TRIP

THE TRIP

Few people like their thunder taken from them,
but even fewer are willing to admit their weakness
and vulnerability during a thunderstorm in life.

Gravel - Smooth Asphalt

A road is often used as a metaphor for life's journey. Life can be smooth or rough, even full of potholes at times. We make life decisions at every fork in the road. Will a person be willing to take the road less frequently traveled when necessary? I liken Mental Illness and Mental Health to gravel compared to a smooth road, partly because of my many years of long-distance cycling on recumbents.

When in apparently stable Mental Health, the road is smooth. That doesn't mean there are no stop signs, hills, or challenging kinds of weather to endure, but the basic surface upon which life is rolling is more or less smooth. A relapse of a Mental Illness is like riding on gravel. Everything becomes more unstable, even grinding one to a halt. If you try to continue rolling on, life is filled with uncertainty, anxiety, and fear. A person with a Mental Illness can fall, and fall fast. Breakdowns of all types are possible - physically, emotionally, and spiritually. You can get scraped up and bruised, and healing takes a long time. The worst-case scenario is severe injury and even death.

Where the metaphor breaks down is that a cyclist on gravel or too rough a road might make a quick correction to get back onto smooth road. Such a correction with a Mental Illness, by contrast, is neither quick nor easy. It can take days, months, perhaps years of diligence, perseverance, and others' assistance to smooth out life's journey and rejoin the regular flow of life, if one is so fortunate.

My experience with cycling has helped me immensely. It is my main place of solitude, prayer, and physical exercise. But it is a highly risky sport, given the errors in judgment I could make, to say nothing of the potential danger that automobiles, trucks, and weather pose. But I accept the challenge and the risk, because I feel truly alive when cycling; it is worth all the fatigue of body and mind. It is a test of endurance and assurance. So, I choose to ride the white line, just barely on smooth road with gravel not far to my right and the potential danger of traffic to my left. Some may see this passion as extreme and don't understand, while others support me in my cycling ventures. Few ride with me; I choose to ride alone.

So too with a Mental Illness. There is a choice, choosing to live with a Mental Illness. Many will not understand or empathize, while others will be supportive. But no one lives the Mental Illness but you. In remission at the moment, I can now say with some assurance, that riding the "right line" of a Mental Illness is worth it. Staying in the smooth lane of life, while acknowledging the reality of a gravel-induced relapse not far off to the right, is worth all the passion and endurance one can muster.

> Closets of life sometimes contain the
> stuff we wish not to admit to and items
> we just as soon not wear in public.

Hide - Run

Run towards something, purposefully. There is a component of motion, of activity, to Mental Health. There is a purpose. When I have a relapse, I tend to try to escape or deny due to anxiety, and then hide due to depression. When I was in an outpatient treatment program, one participant had the fight version of the "fight or flight response" with anxiety, while I have the flight tendency. Instead of getting it all out, I keep it all inside. Eventually if prolonged enough, depression sets in for me. The lack of motivation and even motion in general, as previously described as listlessness of mind, body, and spirit, sets in.

To nurture this in remission and counteract it in relapse, I have learned to run purposefully towards something, typically in a variety of ways. Developing these "running" habits while in remission has given me more tools and skills to deal with a relapse. It has taken me 30+ years of trial and error, and wisdom acquired along the way, to figure out what works for me. Later in the book, in The Modalities section, I will describe the personal ones in more detail. They include exercise, mindfulness, light therapy, proper nutrition, and medication. Here I will describe the journey I have taken to gain some knowledge and self-awareness about their benefits to my Mental Health.

During my most recent relapse and later remission, exercise has been my most consistent private practice. Medication was introduced early, and has changed over time. It involves trial and error with professional help to fine tune what medication or medications are effective. Medication therapy certainly requires patience and pragmatism. With the pattern of relapses occurring almost exclusively during winter, Seasonal Affective Disorder therapy was added to the mix, consisting of Vitamin D, natural light from the sun, and light therapy. I have learned to embrace all of these as vital to my Mental Health.

In addition, in the six years since my first inpatient treatment, I have learned to run towards and appreciate mindfulness, stretching, and nutrition. Both mindfulness and stretching have become part of a near daily ritual for me. More complex, but no less important, is nutrition, which includes food as well as supplements. While I find perfection with nutrition unrealistic, I firmly believe in the motto, "If you put garbage in, don't be surprised if you get garbage out." I cannot address the effects of alcohol, caffeine, or nicotine, as I have never smoked or drunk either coffee or alcohol.

Finally, I have come to appreciate deeply the presence and impact of loving individuals in my life. An entire segment of this book is devoted to this topic. Unfortunately, that realization has been rather late in my journey. Partly this is because I am an introvert, but for everyone, Mental Illness can be a lonely journey that few can even partially comprehend from the outside. The presence of loved ones remains critical nonetheless. Developing and maintaining solid interpersonal relations is essential while in remission, so that I have loved ones to run to for assistance and a loving embrace when a relapse occurs.

I have learned the hard way, a number of times, that a lax attitude to these factors in my Mental Health is an unwise risk. Experience has taught me to keep them tuned up and running while in remission, and to run towards them when a relapse occurs.

Passenger - Driver

Dealing with a lifelong Mental Illness also involves a daily reality. The analogy of a trip each day in a car with a passenger and driver has meaning for me. Later in this book you will read a specific story shared during a group session, which the title of this chapter comes from. I have given my passenger a name, Andy, which stands for <u>An</u>xiety & <u>D</u>epression dail<u>y</u>. Your Mental Illness will be a passenger each day in some way. The question is whether you will remain the driver, or whether instead your Mental Illness will take control of the wheel.

As the previous chapter showed, as long as I try to escape, deny, or hide from my Mental Illness, the illness will be a driving force in my life. A healthier approach, which I had at first thought counterintuitive, even ridiculous, was to befriend Andy. At the time, I thought of my Major Depressive Disorder, Andy, as my mortal enemy, certainly nothing to be chummy with. But today I have come to accept Andy as a passenger for life. I don't have to like it, but it is and will be a part of who I am for life, so I might as well get acquainted with it. I have come to dispense with the woulda, coulda, shouldas, and the guilt and even shame that I may have associated with Andy. Now there is no more hiding or denying that I have a Mental Illness. While Andy is not a badge of honor to wear, I will fight like hell to live an honorable life with Andy. Even in the relapse that occurred two weeks ago, when Andy tried to take the wheel, I needed all my self-driven skills to remain the driver for the majority of those two weeks. It was difficult and brutal mentally, emotionally, and physically, but I was resilient enough to keep at least one hand on the wheel.

My self-driven skills were mentioned in the previous chapter, and I will only claim what has proven helpful for me. Each person must find their own way with their Mental Illness. But this automobile analogy works for me. I had better check that my tires are fully inflated, the oil level is proper, and that regular maintenance is performed on the vehicle. Why? Because my safety is in play; indeed, my life may depend on driver performance. Preparation and diligence, necessary in automobile safety, are necessary as well when living with a Mental Illness. Becoming lax in either is imprudent.

But realize also that enjoyment of your daily trip, even with a Mental Illness, is possible. Yes, I have had to adapt, spend a lot of time on my skills, and realize I will have relapses in my Mental Health. But joy is attainable, is worth surviving relapses for, and is worth sharing with others, even Andy. While sadly this is not so for some with a Mental Illness, I consider myself fortunate and blessed to still be driving each day.

> Choosing a marathon is not the issue, the issue
> is how to prepare oneself to survive one.

Sprint - Marathon

You may think from reading this segment so far, that I am a marathon type of guy. You would be partially right, as I am on a lifelong journey with a Mental Illness. The tortoise wins the race over the hare, right? Steady, persistent diligence will win this Mental Illness marathon. Especially when in remission, this has been true for me, as I have described. The between portion of living with a Mental Illness involves a relapse, when symptoms become so severe that a sprint comes into play.

This type of sprint does not mean adding to the exhaustion of the Mental Illness symptoms, however. As I have experienced many times, fear, panic, and desperation are not helpful. Yes, just as Andy will try to take the wheel, Andy will also pull me into that type of rat race. Besides exhausting me, it will shock and scare loved ones as well. I must remember that the brain that is in dis-ease is still what is needed, even in diminished capacity, to deal with a relapse. There will be moments in a relapse when things are a bit calmer, calm enough to process and think more clearly. Exactly during these moments is when I must quickly assess my situation and plan how to proceed. Then I adjust the plan given the circumstances each day or two, as circumstances warrant.

This type of sprint involves rallying all the methods, skills, and resources available with a plan in mind. Since I just went through a two-week relapse, I will describe this sprint and what worked, at least this time. As symptoms surfaced and became more prevalent, I first told my wife, Rita. Next, I contacted my psychiatrist, in case symptoms became severe enough to warrant Electro-Convulsive Therapy (ECT), and to get advice on medication modifications. As we were within a week of leaving for a warmer and sunnier climate, Rita and I discussed whether we should still go or stay home. We decided to go on the trip with family, knowing that I was only a plane ride away from home and from more invasive ECT treatment if necessary.

So, the sprint as I call it took place. I rallied the methods and human resources necessary. My wife and the psychiatrist became involved. A close friend and my children were aware of the situation in time for additional support. I began taking a small dose of medication for sleep at night, to minimize the exhaustion of the daily symptoms. While on vacation, I walked 2-3 miles upon rising every morning. I got outside in the sun and fresh air as much as possible. I stretched/meditated for an hour each day. I ate healthy food, and very little junk food or processed sugar.

It took a week at home and then one week on vacation before the symptoms faded. It was difficult, brutal, and painful to go through. Rita would attest to this and to how difficult it was for her as well. I do not try to figure out what was the "magic bullet or sauce" that allowed me to go back into remission. But I do know that if I would not have sprinted towards all those methods and resources, I may not have recovered without ECT treatments.

THE LOVED ONES

> When you can't trust yourself, be vulnerable
> enough to trust your friends.

Foe - Friend

Realizing that loved ones will stand by, sit with, and drive me to the hospital when necessary, goes way beyond an ah-hah moment. I have needed both time and events to realize that there are a few exceptional persons who will stick with me through thick and thick. Yes, they even walked through the locked doors of an inpatient psych ward just to be present to my scattered being. They include my wife Rita, my daughters, and other family and friends. The list is not long; I can count them on two hands. I am grateful every time I think about this; often a tear comes to my eye. I have been truly blessed. Most everything about a Mental Illness is a lonely process, but I do not have to survive it completely alone.

But what may be surprising is that loved ones have also been foes in my journey with a Mental Illness. I have come to expect no better or worse from them than I do from anyone who does not know me well. Loved ones typically wish to assist in such an urgent manner, that unfortunate things have been done and said in the name of their love for me. They also typically do not know enough about Mental Illness to offer wise guidance.

Some have said that if my wife were there more to ease my load, things would be better. One was worried that what I was going through was going to tarnish their reputation. One wondered whether it was a trial from God. Others were simply missing from all the action — a deafening silence from them. I do not blame or even need to forgive them. I have come to believe that they did the best they could. They have individual shortcomings and flaws, just as I have. I simply hold up and cherish the handful or two of true friends who were truly present amid my Mental Health crises.

> Feeling sorry for and feeling sorry with
> someone are two vastly different things.

Sympathy - Empathy

The most common responses I have experienced is people feeling sorry for me or nervous "I don't know what to say". There are loved ones who have come close to truly understanding the reality of my Mental Illness. But there are other loved ones, who for whatever reason, would just as soon be a mile away from any contact or recognition of my Mental Illness.

I will never claim that I truly can empathize with another person's Mental Illness. I have only a partial understanding of their situation, even after reflecting on what I have gone through personally. Certainly, I cannot claim to know how they feel, much less share in those feelings. So, I do not expect loved ones to be able to truly empathize with my situation. In fact, I dislike it most when they claim or think that they do.

The best approach loved ones can take with me is honesty and transparency. Those who have come closest to empathy have made it clear that they neither understand what I am going through nor know how I feel. I respect them for being honest. The mind, especially a disease of the mind, is so complex that to state anything else would be a bit arrogant.

So, I will now turn to approaches that loved ones can take. What can they do when they cannot fully understand the emotional turmoil and havoc that a relapse can wreak on my being?

There is a knowing that comes with deep
caring that transcends just understanding
that someone is not well.

Knowledge - Knowing

Whoa! The last chapter was not just brief, it was a bit blunt. Yes, even loved ones cannot totally understand a Mental Illness and certainly can't share in your feelings. But loved ones can learn about Mental Illness generally, and even how it might be manifesting in their loved one who has a Mental Illness. From that base of knowledge, they might begin to partially understand. But note the cautious, humble language. No one has a firm grasp of even a loved one's individual situation. Realize that the mind is very complex.

If you try to care for a loved one without a base of knowledge to work from, it would be like expecting a result from grasping at fog. The temptation is to fill that fog in with something: fear of the unknown, frustration over no quick or easy answers, or even anger at a loved one's condition. Early on a therapist told me, "Mick, it would be a lot easier if you had an eyeball sticking out of its socket." Any relatively hidden illness would be similar, like chronic back pain, which I also live with most days. I wake up and think, "Back by unpopular demand." But to everyone else I seem to walk around and function normally. The danger here is the same; instead of nodding a bit with some understanding, loved ones with no knowledge base are left shaking their heads, shrugging their shoulders, rolling their eyes, crying out of care and frustration, or just walking away.

So, this segment will contain information on Mental Illness generally, which we might then fine tune it towards our loved ones. But such knowledge - "knowing"; it will be partial at best. I don't even know everything about my own Mental Illness, nor will I expect ever to know it all. If we approach a Mental Illness with the aim of figuring it out once and for all, we will be disappointed. I have fallen into this trap myself more than once. This can be maddening, as it feels like any solid footing has been lost.

As I mentioned in The Trip segment, this knowledge is not a destination but a journey. The best we can do is map the next course, while expecting the need for course corrections along the way. That is where what I call knowing comes in. A loved one knows that the person they care about with a Mental Illness may have done everything well, yet they still may have a relapse. They know the course of a Mental Illness is unpredictable. They know that the loved one will need to manage their Mental Illness for life; controlling a Mental Illness is not a realistic goal. There will be bad days ahead, including for loved ones. If a relapse occurs, it is rally, compassion, and diligence time, for they know a crisis may not be far away. Knowing is wisdom acquired over time.

You can be completely alone while at the
same time you are surrounded by others.

Absence - Presence

Loved ones have their own lives and concerns beyond what is going on
with my Mental Health. So, I don't concern myself with their absence,
especially during a relapse when I already have more than enough to
deal with. Beyond their absence for their own issues with life, they
could be absent related to my health condition. Reasons for this absence
could include fear, disbelief, and a sense of inadequacy.

Fear or the apprehension of the unknown is understandable, given
the often hidden and unspoken nature of Mental Illness. Add the
stigmas often associated with Mental Illness such as sanity, trust, and
safety, and I wouldn't blame anyone for wanting to keep even a loved
one at arm's length. There might also be denial or disbelief; *it can't really
be that bad, can it? Maybe it's a momentary thing and will just go away in a little
while. After all, everyone has rough patches in their life.* Finally, the feelings
of inadequacy, being uncertain what to say or do for a loved one, may
make a person shy away from engaging the situation.

I recognize now, from those who came during the relapses I have
had, that it takes nonjudgmental love and fortitude even to show up.
My own loved ones might have found me at home, crouched against
a wall crying, collapsing on a sofa in need of help at a friend's house,
at the emergency room, or at an inpatient Mental Health ward in the
hospital. Yes, seeing a person you know well in such desperate shape

takes some guts. But I think that unconditional love and compassion for me has allowed those loved ones to enter and be present.

Some of those loved ones said a few things, others asked compassionate questions. They didn't state empty platitudes like, "It will be OK," or "Everything works out in the end." They may even claim that they didn't do anything. Wrong! They were present. As corny as it sounds, their presence is the present. To show up, with no intention of fixing anything, and maybe even not saying anything, is invaluable. It is the one gift to a person with a Mental Illness that is the beginning, with maybe no ending, that is priceless.

THE MODALITIES

Being a Pill - Taking a Pill

Medication, when necessary, is a piece of the Mental Health puzzle, though not the entire puzzle. Later I will discuss my experiences with medications, but here I will set the boundaries that I accept with regard to medication. These boundaries are either self-imposed or a function of our culture's views regarding Mental Illness and medication.

I have concerns with taking medication, including the type of medication, dosage, side effects, dependence, and duration of usage. My increasing frustration with the side effects of my main medication six years ago contributed to my slow discontinuance of the medication, while continuing with another medication I only took during the winter. As careful as I was in coming off the medication, I severely relapsed six years ago; this led to inpatient hospital stays over a three-year period, along with discovering the appropriate dosage of a new medication.

More recently I have struggled with dependence, an issue that may be a factor with many medications that are prescribed for the Mental Health issues. Coming off these medications has not been easy and is fraught with risk. My brain was used to, if not altered to depend on, the medication for proper functioning. Therefore, I asked my psychiatrist the dependency question. While not directly answering my concerns with the addictive qualities of the medications, he described it as a matter of tolerance. Was I tolerating the medication well? And if so, what risk was I willing to take in not being covered by such a medication to assist with my Mental Health? In other words, if the remission wheel wasn't broken, don't try to fix it. I concluded that the risk was too high, because I had gone down that path once before, with devastating results. Medication has become a piece of my Mental Health puzzle that I don't fiddle with lightly. Transparency with my wife, along with professional guidance by my psychiatrist is essential when it comes to medication. I take a pill instead of risking being a pill.

The other set of boundaries a person using medication functions within is our culture's views on Mental Illness and medication. I can only claim what I have dealt with myself and what I have heard from others. Mental Illness is complex, and is all too often treated disparagingly and even cruelly at times by others and society at-large. Along with disbelief, there even can be a sort of shaming that occurs towards those having a Mental Illness. After all, one should be able to handle this all by themselves with a little hard work, faith, spine, or whatever else is thrown in to make up the magic elixir of "pulling oneself out of it." In particular, resorting to taking medication for a Mental Illness is seen by many as some sort of failure, with its cousin, pill shaming, not far behind. I simply ignore such attitudes by others now, and believe I have an organic imbalance in my brain chemistry due to a complex set of reasons, that is helped by taking medication. Others may "be a pill" about my medication use for my illness, but I will continue my pill use as a part of my Mental Health.

"Stay out of the middle aisles of the grocery stores."-
My Inpatient Mental Health Ward Psychiatrist

Dead Food - Live Food

When I worked for a small nonprofit Social Service Agency that had a food shelf, we used to call highly processed food "dead food". With our current nutritional knowledge, based on scientific studies, it should be no surprise that too much refined sugar, salt, saturated fats, and preservatives are not good for a person's health. By contrast, foods that come the closest to how they occur in nature are the healthiest. I call this "live food".

One of my wife's common sayings is, "Everything in moderation." There is much wisdom in that statement generally. But Mental Illness is one area where we should lean more towards what my inpatient psychiatrist said to me, "Stay out of the middle aisles of the grocery stores." There is a general concept that if you feed too much garbage food in, don't be surprised if you get garbage out. But with regard to Mental Health, there are neurotransmitters that include serotonin, dopamine, norepinephrine, and gamma-aminobutyric acid (GABA), that affect mood and sense of well-being. Having too much or too little, in other words, an imbalance of these neurotransmitters in your system, can contribute to the type of brain chemistry imbalances associated with Mental Illness.

Your body makes those neurotransmitters, and the building blocks for them come from the food you eat. Recently, I have started looking into those building blocks. As a result, I have added them as supplements to my diet, to make sure I get an adequate amount of the building blocks, along with the good food that I eat. One example is serotonin. I am on an SSRI medication (selective serotonin reuptake inhibitor) for my Mental Illness. Basically, the medication assists in increasing the serotonin in the brain by making it "hang around" longer. So, my thinking went something like this, "If I am taking something artificial to affect the serotonin in my brain, it is prudent to make sure I have enough of the building blocks for serotonin in the food and supplements that I take as well.

> Taking the time and calming oneself long
> enough to accept and befriend one's
> reality is a worthwhile discipline.

Mindless - Mindful

I was a hamster on a hamster wheel once; I am less so now. That hamster-like, mindless behavior lacks any qualities of true processing and reflection of one's life. My thoughts would simply run wild, and I would gravitate towards whatever thought or thoughts were winning on any given day. This pattern becomes especially problematic when I relapse or have symptoms that mimic a relapse. For instance, as I am writing this chapter, I am having trouble differentiating the symptoms of a partial relapse from the symptoms of moderate inner ear vertigo that I may be experiencing. Am I having one or both at the same time? The unsteadiness, slight dizziness, and a bit of nausea that I have had with moderate vertigo are too similar to the anxiety component of a Mental Health relapse that I have experienced. My thoughts will race more than a bit, and my thoughts will gravitate towards the "oh no" of a relapse and its accompanying fear, frustration, and edginess.

Mindfulness is accepting what is happening for what it is, nothing more and nothing less. Thoughts are not real; they will come and go. Whether one calls it mindfulness, meditation, self-awareness, or prayer, I have come to practice it with some success. Later in the book I explain how I practice this. For now, I will say that it has allowed me some sense of space and peace, even while experiencing symptoms. My thoughts can and will get out of control, but the breathing practice I use allows me a brief retreat from those thoughts. I accept what is happening as real and attempt to add no further thoughts. I try to slow my mind down and breathe. As the quote above suggests, I befriend myself as well as my experience in the moment. This is much easier said than done. It takes practice when healthy, so it can be drawn upon when symptoms occur.

From the fishing and bicycling trips I have been on, gentle running water has been a frequent enough occurrence that I can easily imagine myself sitting by a stream or lakeshore as I settle into my breathing. The waves or ripples on the water form the foundation of my breathing from which I observe the coming and going of my thoughts, always able to return to the rhythm of breathing if I become too distracted. The secret or goal of mindfulness practice is to honor and respect yourself and the moment you are in. In doing so some space develops, so you can exist without harsh judgment or ridicule; you give yourself permission to be imperfect and still loved.

Embracing the fatigue and pain is just as true in a
Mental Illness as in physical exercise, that is one reason
physical exercise is a component of Mental Health.

Wiped Out - Exercise

Sound mind sound body, as the saying goes. I need no further proof of the benefits of exercise for Mental Health than what I have seen in my own life. I became convinced of this one winter, some 30 years ago, when I was able to go bicycling. It was the only period of time that I felt normal in my skin, and it would last for a couple hours after each bike ride. To this day, walking and cycling have been part of my daily or weekly routine to not only keep me physically but also mentally engaged. Combined with an almost daily stretching routine, my exercise keeps me engaged and pliable both physically and mentally.

It may sound daunting, but a routine of stretching and exercise forms the backbone of my health. It is especially, even critically important during the winter, when I also struggle with Seasonal Affective Disorder. And surprisingly, I found ways to exercise even when I was hospitalized twice for Mental Illness. Having objectives and goals helped me to be as engaged in the process as possible, in a sense earning the right to be discharged and go home. The exercise I do is deliberate and regular, but not to the point of total exhaustion or being wiped out. Steady, low impact, walking and bicycling sharpens my mind as well as keeping my body tuned up.

While I can easily imagine maintaining my Mental Health without this pill or that pill, I cannot see fighting against a Mental Illness without a healthy lifestyle that combines both healthy eating and exercise.

Answers - Avenues

In my Mental Health journey, I used to look for answers. But now, in the light of my experiences over the past 30+ years, I will take all of the avenues I can get in order to maintain my Mental Health. Early on, like many individuals, I expected that a certain pill and dosage was the long-term solution to my brain chemistry imbalance. Now I view my situation with more complexity and nuance. Now I look for avenues, for opportunities, to aid my Mental Health. In dealing with SAD, chronic back pain, and a family history of depression, the more avenues I explore, the more likely I will maintain good health.

So, I consider all these approaches, with the knowledge that easy answers will be in short supply. Proper nutrition and sufficient exercise are factored in. Light therapy is added for the winter months to help with SAD. I am not opposed to taking a pill or two to help offset my brain chemistry imbalances. Finally, when necessary and as a last resort, ECT has proven helpful in getting my brain back to functioning normally when it relapses.

I believe that a multi-faceted, multi-disciplinary approach gives me the greatest chance of long-term success. Given the complexity of the brain and the many factors that can impact one's Mental Health, I have found that I must employ "all hands on deck" and "leave no stone unturned" strategies, in order to have a reasonable chance of maintaining Mental Health.

REALIZATION

For me, having a significant Mental Illness for over 30 years has not been a dark love story, but it certainly has been about loving the darkness in my life.

You can be an expert in Mental Health, but
know nothing of the experience of Mental
Illness. Experience is the master teacher.

Expertise - Experience

I didn't set out to get well versed in Mental Health, but over more than 30 years, my experience has been a master teacher. What started out as situational anxiety and depression due to chronic pain, quickly morphed into how personal and visceral my walk with Mental Health would become. Experience has provided clues I can garner, as to both how one's Mental Health can deteriorate and practices that help foster Mental Health.

I cannot accurately describe someone else's Mental Health journey, nor can they describe mine. But our shared experience can provide a basis of solidarity around Mental Health, and an openness to deeply listen amidst the pain and suffering of Mental Illness symptoms. From my experiences amidst group sessions with professionals and patients alike, it has become clear that the purest gift we can give is willingness to listen to each other's pain.

Desperation - Perspiration

You gotta put in the hard work. There are few if any shortcuts. Looking honestly at your situation and the multitude of factors involved is indeed hard work. It requires a willingness to be vulnerable and open to outside critique.

Hopeless – Hope

There is a choice during a relapse. Either you are one day more into a violent storm in life or one day closer to the skies clearing.

Why - Wisdom

The trails to why or why me have no end.

The road to loving yourself even with a Mental Illness is the proper destination.

From the Movie – One Flew Over the Cuckoo's Nest

McMurphy *(Jack Nicholson)*:

"What do you think you are, for Chrissake, crazy or somethin'? Well you're not! You're not! You're no crazier than the average a★★hole out walkin' around on the streets and that's it."

ONE FLIGHT INTO THE CUCKOO'S NEST

Acknowledgments 53
Introduction: My "Feelings" of "Andy" 55

SECTION 1: THE FLIGHT

Baggage 61
Passport– Mental Illness IDs 66
Boarding Security– Belt and Shoelaces Please 71
Cocktails and Snacks– The Medications – Educated Guesses 74
Flight Manuals and Magazines– The Programs –
Acronyms Abound - EBT, DBT, CBT etc. 78
Barrel Roll Maneuver - ECT– Not Your
Garden Variety Seizure 81
No Shortage of Other Flights– The Warriors –
The Worn and Weary 85

SECTION 2: PASSENGERS ALONG ON MY FLIGHT

Wife/Lifelong Partner – Rita 91
Daughter – Teresa 95
Daughter - Katie 98
Mother - Lorraine 101
Friend - Gordy 102
Friend – Peter 109

SECTION 3: THE TOUCH DOWN AFFECTION
FOR THE AFFLICTED - WHY KEEP FLYING

The Reaction– "You are No Good to Us Dead" 115
The Recognition– Only the Shadow Knows 118
The Reality– Mental Health Spectrum 121

Body– Show up – Faith 124
Mind– Listen – Hope 127
Spirit– Divine Spark – Love 130

SECTION 4: LIFESAVERS

Dedication

To all the warriors who have personally fought, fight currently, or who lost their earthly lives fighting their Mental Illness.

ACKNOWLEDGMENTS

While my opinion and critique of the Mental Health system is evident in this book, it does not mitigate or extinguish my respect for the capable and diligent mental health professionals of all types from whom I have benefited.

Also, individuals, patients if you will, that I experienced and learned from in in-patient and out-patient settings, have and continue to make a deep impact on my soul. As the dedication alludes, they are whom I consider the true warriors of the subject(s) at hand.

Finally, not everyone will stand nonjudgmentally and empathetically in the pain and dysfunction of your Mental Illness. Twenty-five years ago, I could name them easily on just over one hand. Now as my family, those few friends, and my openness about my illness has grown, I cherish my blessed dozen or so who showed up, in particular, during my in-patient hospital stays in Mental Health units.

It was and continues to be a lonely affair, but I am not alone.

INTRODUCTION

My "Feelings" of "Andy"

I started using the term "Andy," as in <u>A</u>nxiety, <u>D</u>epression, dail<u>y</u>, a couple years ago at age 60, 30 years into my illness and just removed from three in-patient hospital stays and two out-patient treatment programs in four months. But I shall not get too far ahead, as the introduction to the subject, much less my personal reality, of Mental Illness requires reflection on the past.

When I grew up in the 60s and early 70s in my hometown of Hastings, MN near the Twin Cities, stereotypes of those with Mental Illness, and collateral damage done to others using language quips and clichés, were abundant. I was very familiar with words such as "nuts," "loco," "crazy," "insane," or "psycho." Phrases such as "looney bins," "a few French fries short of a Happy Meal®" or "not dealing with a full deck" were used to make fun of the "normal" as well as "those not quite right upstairs".

While I experienced, and bantered around myself, in such terms and phrases to kid around with friends and perceived enemies, Hastings had a Mental Health facility that opened as the 4th MN State Mental Health Asylum in 1900. By 1937, it was Hastings State Hospital, a quite large and mysterious complex deep in the woods off the Vermillion River, with their iconic blue buses that were seen going to and fro occasionally. In gest usually, off the rails behavior might invite someone to yell, "better watch out or the blue bus will come to get ya". In looking up

Hastings State Hospital history, I was pleased to see that it was often innovative in the state system for things such as discontinuing using restraints and starting chemical addiction programs. Mental Illness and how individuals were "committed", much less treated, was one mystery of my youth.

In 1975, the iconic film *One Flew Over the Cuckoo's Nest* came out, the same year I graduated from High School. It swept the top five Oscar awards that year and has been named on the short list of most culturally significant movies ever made. With its comedic and sadistic stew, the book made into a movie tells the tale of the duel between the inflexible head of the psych ward, buxom nurse Ratched, and the cocky new patient seeking a lighter environment than a prison farm, Randle McMurphy. Told through the voice of long-term patient, Chief Bromden, constraints and restraints are the norm, along with prolific use of drugs to keep patients under control. Ultimately, electroshock therapy, a suicide, a lobotomy, and the mercy killing of McMurphy by Bromden brings the movie to a sad climax.

Looking back now, in a short eleven+ years after High School, and health that youth assumes, I would then begin my own flight through the cuckoo's nest. It is true that everything cuckoo's nest has changed in the past 40-50 years, much for the better, but much still needs to be addressed as well. While touching lightly on my 30+ year journey with "Andy" (I wrote a book titled *Bicycle Built for the Blues* for this), the following is primarily based on my last 3+ year experiences with "Andy," which includes now four in-patient hospital stays, two out-patient programs, individual professional counseling, Electroconvulsive Therapy, multiple changes in medication, and long stretches of "Andy" being a minor passenger on my flight of life and not an overbearing pilot. As no one's flight in life, much less with "Andy" is a solo flight, the impact my Mental Illness has had on others is a reality as well. Finally, in my present state of relative stable Mental Health while writing this book, I will address why I am hopeful and what I have found helpful in regard to .

So, are you ready to come fly with me in a flight in the cuckoo's nest?

A promise to myself, as well as you, my thoughts will be
transparent and my feelings will be raw and laid bare.

I have feelings of ANDY
As tears roll down my face
If I would to do over again
Would I choose any other place?

The will to live runs short
As the days seem way too long
A few stand by my side
When they feel something is wrong

Answers seem to run short
In the darkness of ANDY
A "pill" to get used to
Anything but candy

Trying to accept
Andy within my space
When in remission, indeed choose
To accept this place

SECTION ONE

The Flight

My God, my God, why have you forsaken me?
Why are you so far from helping me, and
from the words of my groaning?
My God, I cry in the daytime, but you don't answer;
in the night season, and am not silent.

Baggage

We all have baggage of one sort or another, and while most of us have some baggage we wish we wouldn't have to claim, it is still our baggage. At the risk of that baggage going round and round endlessly, and never truly being picked up and dealt with, we ignore our baggage. The analogy for Mental Health is that I must truly own and deal with all of my baggage, large and small, heavy or light, no matter how disturbing. Some would say through prayer, meditation, and/or counseling, one can lighten the load of such baggage, but my belief is that no one can totally put it down. While I would certainly say I do not like some of my distressing baggage, and will never consider them a friend, they still will be on every flight, on every journey in life I take. To that end, I offer a fair amount of the mental baggage I will carry, hopefully in healthy way, for the remainder of my life.

A Sampling of My Mental Health Baggage – Old to New that I Carry
(A chronology of sorts)

Thirty-four years ago, I woke up one December day to get ready for work and could not turn easily side to side. The frustration and effort to overcome the daily chronic pain that ensued is one of my most visible pieces of baggage marking my life's journey. It brought me out of my first profession as a Dentist, it exhausted me emotionally and spiritually, it brought me literally to my knees.

In Dental practice, I struggled to maintain the quality of my dental work (let's say B+ average) while trashing my emotional/mental wellbeing (enter high anxiety and depression) in the process.

There were many nights, 20-30 years ago, that I would be overcome with emotion and get up out of bed to cry in another room so as not to disturb my wife, Rita.

I changed everything possible in my Dental profession for 10 years to maintain my practice. I eventually settled on only 3-4 hours 3 mornings a week, sort of pretending to still have a practice because I did not see any other option at the time.

I fell to my knees in front of my wife, balling my eyes out and she suggested for the first time that I see a therapist. I remember how I felt, being socially conditioned, when I drove myself in fear and dread to a therapist for the first time and sitting in the waiting room.

The guilt-ridden feelings surfaced, for not being able to hold up my end of the deal as a husband, and a father of two young children.

I would go for lonely walks of only one mile and felt frustrated and dejected that my back ached so much.

I called into a crisis line to discuss having suicidal thoughts but no plan.

After one of my lonely walks, my emotional grip on myself was lost and I experienced my first panic attack and began hyperventilating.

I took the MMPI for the first time while in counseling and was told I was clinically depressed.

I understood that a solution/answer was typically more than one thing, and went to all kinds of specialists looking for an answer: Orthopedic surgeon, Neurosurgeon, Chiropractor, Acupuncturist, Allergist, Osteopaths and Physical Trainer.

After an orthopedic surgeon gave me the option of back surgery, I discovered through the neurosurgeon and patients who had had the procedure, how invasive the surgery would be with only a 50-50 chance of making any improvement in pain.

The neurosurgeon stated quite bluntly that I shouldn't want this type of thoracic back surgery unless I couldn't walk or was peeing on the floor from effects of direct spinal cord impingement.

I was so emotionally stressed while trying to do dentistry near the end, that when I gave a lower mandibular block injection to a patient who flinched, I then flinched as well.

I concluded after suffering in dental practice for 10 years to give up on my profession that I worked so hard to achieve.

My first go-round with antidepressants was Prozac, and I lost 8 pounds in three days due to night sweats. I was giving a little presentation at a staff meeting and could think of what I wanted to say, but could not speak effectively to those thoughts. The ethics of practicing dentistry in such a state dictated to me that I should, and did, discontinue taking Prozac.

The memory is vivid of the conversation I had with my brother and father who I was in dental practice with; I cried when telling them I was giving up Dentistry.

I was fortunate with my first therapist, Mark, who listened through my processing of my family upbringing and decision to give up dental practice. On telling me that through this whole process I had been making good decisions, he said, "Mick, if you told me that your next decision was to go to Nepal and see a guru, and he told you to eat lama shit, I would trust you at this point." I remembered that I laughed and knew that some hope for normalcy had returned.

Etched in my mind forever is the moment I was sitting against a wall in my young daughter Teresa's bedroom to cry after my wife went off to work; she came into the room without my knowing it, put her hand on my shoulder and said, "It will be OK daddy."

In a sort of denial after giving up patient practice, I did some book and HR type work in the basement of the Dental office, pretending I still had a job, since I didn't know what else to do.

After giving up dentistry, and made the decision to go big time into careful physical training to strengthen my back and discovered, while in training, that if I rode a recumbent stationary bike, it did not exacerbate my back pain.

One winter, even after giving up dentistry, I had a critical anxiety attack and told my wife I did not feel safe and that she should call for an emergency county crisis intervention. Two ladies came over, and I remember telling them that "going to the dental office was like going to an accident scene with yellow tape around it." Her answer really stuck, "If it is that bad, then why do you keep going back." I decided to leave the family practice completely shortly thereafter.

The following autumn, I got my first recumbent road bike, a red, long wheelbase, Ryan with under the seat steering, to test out the next spring whether recumbent bicycling would be my one main physical outlet I could do with no back pain.

After going to a specialist who did a myelogram, he told me of four thoracic discs that were ruptured and it made no need to test any further. He told me that I was lucky that I did not have surgery before when the only MRI result then was one herniated disc – that surgical intervention would likely have been a never-ending cascade of increasing back problems and pain.

Finding out what really was wrong with my back, after 10+ years of suffering in pain, felt like a relief. Knowing what I was up against was some comfort.

One tough winter mentally, I biked a few times, at least once each month, when the weather was in the mid-30's and the road shoulders were clear. I had about 2 hours of mental clarity and feeling normal in my own skin. I knew at that point that there was a biochemical possibility of some mental normalcy I could achieve due to this endorphin-type experiment.

I was on my third therapist/psychiatrist when I told her of a seeming winter pattern of emotional turmoil and trouble. She apologized for a diagnosis of SAD, along with depression, never being considered before while in therapy. I then began an antidepressant drug combination (Paxil and Wellbutrin) along with light therapy in the winter.

I felt nearly normal on Paxil for over 15 years. In that relative state of mental health, I changed careers twice, and became a Deacon in the Catholic Church followed by a Master's degree. I increasingly became an avid recumbent cyclist to the extent that I rode in every state, and did 10 fundraising rides over 10 years while raising $100,000 for various charities.

In hindsight, I realized that the riding, including two cross-country rides and Alaska/Yukon, while for enjoyment and altruism, were also to prove something to myself – that I was good enough even amidst the backpedaling I had done in mental health and professional careers.

I was typically more tired and had sexual dysfunction while on Paxil; I did not like the side effects but tolerated them.

The fall of 2016 I decided, without doctor's advice, after being on my typical low dose of summer Paxil, to try getting off Paxil very slowly and just stay/increase Wellbutrin for my usual winter dose.

On December 8th, 2016 while on vacation in Florida and having a great time, I woke up at 3:00 pm for a brief bit with that all too familiar anxiety feeling from the past. It got progressively more pronounced in intensity and duration to the point it was always in the background by the time we flew home from vacation two days later where I went back to work at my job as a Chaplain at my hometown hospital and senior living facility.

It is obvious by now that I have some baggage, a little of which is good, from living with my Mental Illness. There is more baggage, but that will be offered in other portions of this book. To unpack those bags a bit in advance, over the last three years I have had four inpatient stays in two Mental Health units. My medication regimen is completely different, and I have gone through two outpatient therapy programs. Most recently, it made sense to undergo 11 ECT (electroconvulsive therapy) treatments as a way to assist in achieving a healthier and less dire mental/emotional state. My image at the time, although more positively altered now, is that a person does not go into a lockdown Mental Health unit unless things are really, really bad. I now have entered that whispered about, if at all, exclusive club of having a Major Depressive Disorder. It is major, not minor, depressive to the degree of no hope, and I am disordered. Having claimed a fair amount of my baggage from the past, let us depart on my flight in the cuckoo's nest of the last four years.

Passport

Mental Illness IDs

Some mentally charged sayings from my youth I can identify with and echo in my mind now. These include, "You are such a pill," "You're such a pain," and "Are you out of your mind?" A couple things I have learned during my Mental Health journey are that it is important to fully embrace my true identity(ies), including the IDs of my illness(es), and that I risk some peril if I think they have an expiration date.

I remember looking for the silver bullet in my search for the magic answer (or answers) that would make my back disability and consequent pain go away. I equally remember a phase in which I thought having only one or two magic pills to rebalance my brain chemistry would solve my depression, anxiety, and SAD. I view myself much more pragmatically and compassionately now. In retrospect, two comments made by others penetrated my perception of self; one I embraced fully and the other I did not believe, but in hindsight should have.

The first occurred several years into dealing with chronic pain with my back and after I found out I had at least four ruptured thoracic discs along with the advice not to have surgery. Okay, I said to myself, then I am going to learn to strengthen my back through appropriate training and exercise, along with seeking out top expert advice in dealing with the mental component of my pain complex. I followed through with the learning and training, and one winter went through the multi-week chronic pain program at St. Mary's Hospital (Mayo) in Rochester. The very first day of the chronic pain program at Mayo, they emphasized to the group of eight or so of us going through the program that, "You are not your pain." As half of the participants were hooked on one pain medicine or another to escape their pain, I sensed in the group, including myself, that pain had become a (if not the) dominant force in most of our lives. And so, in the program, the physical and mental gymnastics of reducing each individual's dependence on pain pills started while convincing us of our worth and identity separate from pain. I considered myself either lucky or fortunate in comparison. I was not taking any pain medication as I could not ethically consider doing dentistry in an altered state, and I did not have pain to deal with when laying back or lying down. Sleeping well was not an issue, thankfully. Therefore, this concept of not being my pain was much easier for me than for many in the group, as there were stretches of time each day that I did not experience nearly unbearable physical pain. While I learned that the pain was certainly not in my head, I did not sufficiently deal with the mental aspect of the pain, the wear and tear on my Mental Health, and thereby the pain was more or less tolerable depending on how I thought about it and my general state of Mental Health. Physical signs of pain made me heed their warning to pay attention and back off, but the signs of mental distress and dysfunction were not heeded in a similar way. To my demise mentally, I just pushed on.

Enter the second comment concerning mental health, the one I did not embrace totally, but should have in hindsight. In late 1989, after three years of back pain but still doing dentistry on a reduced scale for another seven years, I went to counseling for the first time upon my wife's encouragement and found out from an MMPI test that I was clinically depressed. After taking myself off Prozac due to the side effects, I decided one month later that I would like to enter the three-year formation program to become a Deacon in the Roman Catholic Church. As I pushed on, it is bewildering even to this day why my wife and I entertained a religious formation process at such a crisis-ridden time in our family life. I was slowly losing my sole occupation and we had two small daughters at home.

One step in the approval process for diaconate formation was a psychologist who ran all the candidates and their wives through a battery of psychological tests lasting several hours on a Saturday. Then she met with each of us individually. The psychologist told me bluntly, "Mick, you are a very good candidate for the formation program, but you will need help dealing with your mental health your entire life." As amazing as Rita and my desire was to seek acceptance into the program, equally amazing was the candidate committee, with advice from the psychologist, that let us into the program several months after taking an MMPI that showed I was clinically depressed.

So, I pushed on with long periods of health interrupted by some shorter periods of mental distress and anxiety, especially during the winter months. Along the way, paying attention to Seasonal Affective Disorder (SAD) was added to the mix, and along with seeking psychological and pharmaceutical help, I was mostly stable for 25 years. I had a pretty good thing going: relative health with a certain dosage of antidepressant and some occasional counseling. I exercised often and consistently, and along with taking my "happy" pills to balance my brain chemistry, I thought to myself, "I am just fine – thank you very much." I could look in the mirror and see a person with a trashed back, but I could not see a person with a serious Mental Illness as well. If I had a "Mental Illness passport" it would read, "Mick Humbert" and *"back disability with depressive tendency & SAD"* listed underneath. Certainly, my MI passport would not list a serious Mental Illness. But that would slowly change.

The stamping of my Mental Illness passport had begun; passing ports of no return (every play on words intended). The first was deep scars from giving up Dentistry and many physical activities due to physical pain; **stamp** – *chronic lifelong back pain with depressive tendency and SAD.* Next, I can still remember to this day, driving to, then passing time in the waiting room, as I waited for my first counseling session. There was loss, grief, fear, and coming to grips with needing help; **stamp** – *I need some help as I cannot control this myself.* Next, I see hyperventilating for the first time, and then later calling for the county crisis intervention I mentioned in the previous chapter when having another such episode; **stamp** – *I have lost all control, if not actually having* *a nervous breakdown.* Some 25 years later, having refined my seasonal (increase in winter) cocktail to include Paxil and Wellbutrin, I decided to stay on Wellbutrin during the winter but very slowly get off the very small dose of "summer" Paxil I was on in the early fall of 2016. And yes, I did this with no physician/psychiatrist supervision. As mentioned previously, everything fell apart in early December of 2016 while on vacation. That all-too familiar anxiety feeling, then depression, and a level of numb panic followed over two weeks. I went down, hard and fast.

My next stamp on my MI passport came that December when sitting in my psychologist's office with my wife, bewildered and bawling, as the psychologist recommended going into the hospital. I asked, "What choice do I have?" She stated I had a choice or it would be made for me. Enter passing a significant port of no return. Security shows up to escort you in a wheelchair from the office building to the Emergency Department (of United Hospital in this instance). Along the way, we passed a security guard who also worked in my hometown of Hastings at the hospital where I worked as well. It was shocking seeing him, and I engaged in a bit of self-shaming. After Initial processing, an emergency room, and some MI intake specialists later, my wife and I waited for several hours for an opening in any mental health facility in their system.

A place in the psych ward of United opened up, and I was wheelchaired up to their lowest level risk unit. I entered through the doors of the unit for processing. It had a central small lounge area with the nurse's station to one side. Double rooms circled around the lounge while the TV blared as a few other patients watched. Staff asked for my belt and shoelaces, and the bathroom in the double room was locked until staff felt it safe enough for me to have open privileges. Except for the absence of actual clanging metal doors, I was a prisoner as much as a patient. Rita left, as I watched her walk way through the small windows in the now locked doors. **Stamp** – *I am potentially a harm to myself and others; freedom and choice are a luxury to be denied for everyone's benefit.*

Through this first MI hospital stay, among the roller coaster of emotions, were staff psychiatrist conversations, explanations, tweaking of meds, and the official diagnosis – Major Depressive Disorder. Oh no, not minor, but big, overpowering depression. I am disordered is how I took it. Immediately after this first hospital stay, which lasted over Christmas, I learned that statistically 10% of patients who end up in a psych ward will eventually and successfully commit suicide. Due to my symptoms, new drug regimen, two outpatient programs, and two more hospital stays that winter, a refined diagnosis of Bipolar II was suggested. **Stamp** – *Major league MI with suicidal ideations from anxiety-driven depression.*

My Mental Illness passport has had a couple more stamps since then. Those ports of no return will follow in other chapters of this book. Here I wish to conclude with a common phrase, "You must own your own sh _ _." Yep, I must deal with my shame. In the depth of my being came the tough task of ownership and identity. As I had earlier taken ownership of my physical pain, I needed to take full ownership of a Mental Illness for life as well. If I were to truly own my Mental Illness, the raw and visceral shame, frustration, anger, and self-loathing needed to be conquered by self-respect and self-love. I needed to surrender to my reality.

As I am deadly serious about this next chapter, I
thought I would start with an airport security joke:
A man walks up to the security counter at the
airport holding a dead possum. The attendant
asks "Sir, will you be checking that?"
The man replies "No, it's carrion."

Boarding Security
Belt and Shoelaces Please

Most everyone who has flown on a flight has gone through Boarding Security. Necessary for everyone's safety, it is still a bit degrading, not so much in what they make you do or take off, but in the assumption that no one can be trusted. Here I wish to elaborate on the degrading, if not dehumanizing, aspects of inpatient mental health hospital wards, at least from my experience. I experienced much of what follows at United Hospital in St Paul. Thankfully, I was also at an inpatient ward in Hutchinson that had a much more friendly approach and custom facility to meet the needs of MI patients.

As mentioned previously, there are no shoelaces or belts allowed, and your bathroom is locked as well, until they can trust you. Part of my tendency once I am in the deepest depths of Andy, is that I lose my appetite. By the time I entered the psych ward for the first time, I had lost 10 pounds in just over two weeks. The jeans I was wearing were hanging on me loosely, and my other alternative was the patient scrubs given out. Remember that typically there is no time to pack ahead of time for the flight in the cuckoo's nest. Personal hygiene is fine except they don't allow you to have a bladed shaver. They did have a small cordless shaver that was the equivalent of scraping off facial hair with coarse sandpaper. Only when I got my frequent flyer designation (multiple hospital ward visits) did I learn to bring slippers, and sandals, a decent battery-operated cordless shaver, and ask for 2 zip ties to put through the loops on each side of my pants to make the pants fit more comfortably.

I was in a double room at United. After the first night with my initial roommate, I begged to have a different room. My roommate was fine, but he needed a bariatric bed that kept adjusting air pressure at night continuously, on top of his heavy snoring. When a person is in great mental and emotional distress, and is struggling to deal with themselves, having a roommate and lack of privacy is not ideal in my opinion. If you stay long enough in the unit, as I did, there is a fair likelihood that your roommate will depart, and another will come within a day as there is a severe shortage of Mental Health beds available in the United States. Again, it does not make intuitive sense to me that a person who can hardly stand to be in their own skin has to tolerate the presence of a roommate.

You might ask, why not get out into the public area for a sense of freedom and peace of mind? Mmmm, that is the "crucible" as I call it, for the basic shape of the public space at United Hospital. I understand they put their Mental Health units into an existing round tower structure, but "small and confining" does not do it justice. At the top of the crucible (the neck) was a long table, a public telephone, and a refrigerator and cupboards with supplies. Outsiders could bring you outside food, which is marked with your name, and into a locked refrigerator it goes. You asked to have it unlocked if you wanted something. In the bowl of the crucible was the roughly thirty-foot circle with the double rooms surrounding it. On one half of the circle was another long table for eating and another public telephone (privileges to call out were given only when there was no scheduled programming). The other half had a few sofa-type chairs around a mounted TV on a pillar. All the chairs in the unit are purposely very heavy; you don't want a patient throwing things around. Just enough room was around the outside of the crucible for two people to walk side by side if all the doors to the patient rooms were closed. No or little outside light penetrated the rooms, crucible, or anywhere else in the unit. At the base of the bowl was the nurses' station on one side, and a small conference room with a larger program room behind it. In between at the base was the double locked doors, or escape hatch, depending on whether you were coming in or exiting. Except late at night, the TV was on nearly all the time when no programming was taking place in the crucible. To summarize, I liken the crucible to a good-sized noisy, open concept living and dining room with no windows that holds about fourteen patients 24/7.

Amidst all this, the professional staff – nurses, counselors, psychiatrists, and various program-related personnel – overall do an admirable job with only a few exceptions. But this does not minimize, or alleviate, the structural deficits of such a Mental Health unit. Later in the book I will address my bewilderment, angst, and hope in this regard in comparison with other health issues of equally significant importance and prevalence in American society.

Aah, yes. Mental Health unit boarding security for human safety is also dehumanizing, or at least contrary to mental health, as well. Take away personal comforts - check. Take away privacy - check. Take away any source of outside light - check. Take away a chance at silence most of the time, except at night - check. Take away personal control and independence - check. Take away nearly all ways to get exercise - check. Into the crucible you go, and turn up the flame when a person is already at the boiling point, and see if you survive. Sorry, but sobering and in some ways cruel imprisonment, is what comes to mind.

Cocktails and Snacks

The Medications – Educated Guesses

Treating Andy (anxiety and depression daily) with medications in the American healthcare system seems to be as common as getting a free drink and snack on an airplane. Add a visit or more into the cuckoo's nest, and both the use of and hopefully the sophistication around prescribing them goes up. Why do I say hopefully? Because any prescriber with an ounce of honesty should tell you that the medications, from antidepressant, antianxiety, and antipsychotic meds to sedatives have research behind them and generally have effectiveness, BUT whether a medication will work well for any given individual is an educated guess at best.

What follows is not necessarily scientifically sound or meant to be an overriding critique or endorsement of a certain medication for any individual. It is simply my experience with the triumphs and tragedies of using medications for Andy personally. That is why I used the quote from Aristotle above; knowing yourself and how you react to medications once started, along with honesty around why you are willing or not willing to take medications, forms a source of personal wisdom that should be paid attention to.

I had only been on three medications before entering the cuckoo's nest. As stated before, after losing 8lbs in three days due to night sweats on Prozac along with its effect on clarity of thought and concentration, I took myself off of it as I could not ethically practice dentistry in such an altered state. Then, after several years of trial and error, and the diagnosis of SAD as well, I hit a sweet spot on relatively low dosages of Paxil™ (paroxetine) and Wellbutrin® (bupropion). I was on a very low-maintenance dose of Paxil™ in the summer and would slowly raise it into fall through winter along with adding a low dose of Wellbutrin®. Winters were always an issue more than any other time of year, but I was able to manage with relative stability for about 15 years.

In hindsight, my tragic mistake came in the fall of 2016 when I decided on my own to just eliminate the low dosage of Paxil™ (10mg) that I was on during the summer, since I did not like the sexual dysfunction and other side effects of Paxil™, and continue using only Wellbutrin®. I was extremely careful in going off Paxil™, more cautious than any physician, counselor, or psychiatrist ever started dosages or changed them for me. I am not saying they weren't cautious, I just knew that going on AND off these medications should be treated with great respect.

After the beginning of my hard and fast descent into the familiar realm of high anxiety while on vacation in Florida that December, I asked for a meeting with a local physician within a week of getting home, seeking some medication assistance to right my sinking ship. I also recognized my error and put myself back on Paxil™ at no different dosage or pace than in the beginning. I was somewhere on the spectrum of panic, despair, and desperation and on the physician's advice began taking Buspar (buspirone) while working as a chaplain. Along with my Prozac experience, it was the most disoriented I have felt on medication – like walking in concrete shoes while dizzy while taking all my effort to focus on the smallest tasks of concentration.

As stated earlier in the Passport chapter, I would be admitted for the first time into an inpatient mental health unit within two weeks. The psychiatrist stopped the Buspar and put me on Xanax® (alprazolam) in addition to the Paxil™. Besides the issue, as stated before, that medications are a trial-and-error business, an educated guess at best, many of the antidepressants take weeks to achieve peak effectiveness. So yes, individuals who are anxious and depressed, and sometimes suicidal, have to rely on an educated guess that takes 4-6 weeks to find out if it helps. I recovered a bit and was sent home in 5-6 days and began the partial inpatient program for 3 weeks while not working.

On relatively recent additions of medication, and not anywhere near fully recovered, I relapsed again when I tried going back to work part time and ended up in the ED again, this time transferred to Hutchinson hospital where I was driven by ambulance in a snow storm. During my stay in Hutchinson, with a psychiatrist I ended up having a lot of respect for, we decided to somewhat slowly discontinue Paxil™ and begin on Cymbalta® (duloxetine). Instead of Xanax®, Seroquel® (quetiapine) was also chosen for the anxiety portion of my disorder. The facility was enlightening, literally and figuratively, compared to United Hospital, and I began to stabilize enough to be released after just under a week.

That did not hold, in hindsight because I was not on the Cymbalta® long enough to reach peak performance, along with the negative side effects of coming off Paxil™. I ended up in United hospital again, where I was put on Desyrel® (trazodone), while getting Paxil™ out of my system and remaining on the Cymbalta®. Here's the shocker, literally. A common side effect of coming off Paxil™ is what they call brain zaps. What I felt on occasion several times each day I can only describe as what I have felt the couple of times after I have gotten accidentally shocked while getting my fingers too close to an electrical outlet. Trazodone is of the same drug family (SSRI) as Paxil™ and Cymbalta®. But to no other factor that I can attribute to, when I started on Trazodone my blood pressure collapsed to the near danger zones (~90 over 50). I collapsed in the bathroom one evening and got myself back to bed. Then another evening, I woke up and went to the nurse's desk, at which point I collapsed to the floor. When I woke up staring at attendants and the ceiling, my affect made them wonder whether I had had a seizure. Off to the epileptic floor I went for an entire day's worth of evaluation, the halo electrodes on my head and all. At this point, with brain zaps, Trazodone side effects, and everything else I had gone through in a couple months, I wanted to die. I said as much to my wife Rita and daughter Teresa who were visiting, and the psychiatrist I was assigned to.

No, I did not have a seizure, but with the psychiatrist's help, what was happening with the medications was brought into question and discussed. Trazodone was eliminated, and Paxil™ was finally out of my system. Seroquel® during the night and a smaller dosage during the day was maintained. The psychiatrist had one other suggestion if

I didn't stabilize, that being ECT (Electroconvulsive Therapy). ECT is an improved procedure now, but it still sounded straight out of the Cuckoo's Nest movie at the time. I stabilized after a few more days and was released into the multi-week Day program. At the end of the ward visit, I found out indirectly that due to the shortage of MI beds, there is a regular morning staff meeting with a component being pressure to release patients from care as soon as possible.

I went back to work part-time and then to my regular schedule as chaplain on Cymbalta® 30 mg, and a Seroquel® dosage that changed summer versus winter, while in the care of a psychiatrist for meds and psychologist for therapy. Seroquel® would eventually be reduced to only a night dosage. My 4 months of MI hell and the cuckoo nest visits had ended. Or so I thought. I wrote a book, part poetry and part prose, in the last two days of the third hospital stay and then several weeks afterward. I wanted a record of my thoughts and feelings while in the depths of the MI crisis, not just after reflection on the cuckoo's nest when the flight was a distant memory. I had reached stability of my mental health, which held for two years.

My points of wisdom, for myself, after all of this were:

1. Medications may be necessary to assist in balancing brain chemistry, but they have a mirror image (live-evil) reality; potentially necessary to live well, they also have an evil side too. You take these cocktails at considerable risk.
2. As I exercise, eat well enough, and use light therapy, along with MI-focused vitamin supplements, I had come to the conclusion that I would be on some form of medication my entire life. In other words, doing all the right "other things," would never be enough, mainly during the winter months.
3. There are therapeutic ranges in the doses used with these medications, and my personal experience has been that lower to middle range dosages have been effective for me.

While it is important to consider whether my Andy issues are genetic, back pain, or social/situational in nature, being able to accept the Mental Illness and an effective drug regimen for it is equally important.

Flight Manuals and Magazines
The Programs – Acronyms Abound - EBT, DBT, CBT etc.

A quick check of the pocket in front of your seat on an airplane and you are likely to find the following items:

- Description of the plane and maybe some maps of airplane terminals
- What to do and how to manage an emergency
- Air sick bag
- Assortment of other people's crap and garbage perhaps

In the course of my flight in the cuckoo's nest I was in a three-week Partial inpatient and a multi-week Day program based on Dialectical Behavioral Therapy (DBT), as well as a condensed version of Cognitive Behavioral Therapy (CBT) while an inpatient in the Hutchinson MI Unit. Both made the claim to be Evidence-Based Therapy (EBT); in my words - it has been tried and it can and has worked for anxiety and depressive disorders. I can't tell you the real or subtle differences between the two, although there was no shortage of flight/program manuals with individual and group exercises, theory, explanations, and a bounty of acronyms that I guess are supposed to be catchy and easy to remember. My opinion is that when a person is not in their "wise mind," as promoted in the programs, it seems a bit ridiculous to expect the level of memory and concentration needed to find acronyms themselves useful. Frankly, I don't remember what any of them stood for and my program manuals are in a drawer by my bedside stand collecting dust.

This does not mean I did not learn, absorb, and own a fair amount of good information. The material was thoroughly and professionally presented by two or three therapists/instructors/pilots. Like flight instructions on the airplane, I listened with a lot of other distractions going through my mind. I absorbed and owned bits and pieces that proved useful. The main blocks of Mindfulness, Interpersonal Effectiveness, and Emotional Regulation had nuggets of good information on how to positively deal with my current mental emergency. Along with my direct and indirect education and knowledge from my own life, the program affirmed a lot of what I knew already. So yes, for me there was a wee bit of learning, good affirmation of known concepts, and a fair amount of "oh, I have heard this all before."

However, within the formal programming, I found the topic of Distress Tolerance (aka - air sick bag) the most compelling because I was in mental and emotional distress. Useful were the suggestions of how to assess and pull back from the white-knuckle syndrome when the mental flight gets bumpy, along with physical skills/tricks such as deliberate breathing techniques and cold-water shock treatment. While I had used mindfulness breathing/meditation before for my back pain, I started to use it when my mind was similarly stressed. The shock of a very cold shower did shock my system enough to allow some temporary relief. During the cuckoo's nest period of severe distress, despair, and depression, I took plenty of cold showers – as in the colder the better-make you shudder audibly – type of showers.

Most importantly, the group sessions with a therapist, and the insights and challenges addressed in them, proved for me the most profound aspect of the programs. I believe dealing with my own crap and garbage in an open nonjudgmental setting, as well as listening and compassionately discussing other people's garbage and crap has been one essential component of my recovery. I showed some anger and cried in front of others in telling and grappling with my own reality, as I witnessed anger, fear, and tears from others as well.

As a matter of confidentiality, I will never share the conversations held within the group sessions or the personal reality that individuals were dealing with. But one of my most memorable and influential discussions revolved around the idea/concept a therapist brought up. She advised that we needed to make friends with our disorder, and she wasn't kidding. I couldn't believe it and argued against what sounded to me like pure nonsense (I'll spare you the more colorful language I used). I had already come to grips with the reality that I would be cursed with this disorder my whole life, but to cozy up and make friends with it?! At that moment, I saw my disorder as an enemy, as a matter of life and death, not as a BFF.

As the steam stopped coming out of my ears, the second comment she made started to make more sense. "Your disorder will be a passenger and along for the ride your whole life, but you are the driver. You don't have to like it, but you need to get up close and intimate with your disorder in order to learn how to keep it from becoming the driver of your life." I had done this with my chronic back pain, and slowly started accepting the wisdom in doing so with my Mental Illness as well. Yes, I now call my disorder, Andy.

> Is it like a reboot for the brain?
> Does it especially target the mood centers of the brain?
> I don't care if it's not completely understood,
> I just know it has helped me when in relapse tremendously.

Barrel Roll Maneuver - ECT
Not Your Garden Variety Seizure

I was mistakenly on mental health autopilot, along with being back to work, when in 2018, while on vacation again in early December, a slower version of the anxiety feeling arose again. Coming back from vacation, I immediately made "my team" aware of what was going on as the feeling became more intense. I started in the Partial inpatient program again within a few days. Of course, "Oh no, here we go again, AGAIN," swirled around in my head. I went down hard and fast again and could not get myself to drive to the program by the end of the first week. Basically, I wept against the floor of the bathroom after taking a shower and told Rita I needed to go to the hospital. Rita drove me up to United where we talked with the nurse of the program, and after an ED visit, I ended up in United again – first in a higher risk unit, and when a room opened up within a day, back to the unit I had been in before.

Coincidence, serendipity, providence, or good luck put me with a roommate who was beginning to go through Electroconvulsive Therapy (ECT). I was able to ask him about the procedure and saw him after he had gone through a couple of the procedures. I eventually asked the psychiatrist on the unit, the same one I'd had before in the winter of 2016/2017, about ECT. They then have you watch a video about the procedure, followed by a psychiatrist-to-psychiatrist consult with my specialist on the "outside." After their input, my praying about it, and talking it over with Rita, I decided to go for the "barrel roll maneuver," as I call it for this book. To put as simply as I can, ECT involves having a brain zapped for a few seconds to induce a seizure. They explained how the procedure had improved in the last 40 years, especially those areas that affect mood and emotions. The description sounded like a sophisticated reboot of the brain. Yes, they were honest in stating they don't know all the why's of why it works on some people; they just know that it does.

Fortunately, as well, my "outside" psychiatrist was one of three that does the procedure at United. Along with an increase in my dosage of Cymbalta®, I was set up for several ECT procedures while in the hospital. If effective, I would be released home to complete the remaining of the full series (11 total) ECT treatments on an outpatient basis. In my case, the time between ECT treatments would be increased as the series progressed. I also knew from my team, as well as reading up a bit, that some individuals go in for "maintenance" treatments as needed.

For the barrel roll maneuver itself, and how hard it might be to consider turning your brain upside down to the point of a seizure, I can say I was nervous but not apprehensive about the procedure ahead of time. As stated before, I had seen and talked to my roommate a couple times after his procedures before he was released from the cuckoo's nest. Typical to any procedure with light anesthesia, I did not eat anything after supper the day before. When time came for my first ECT, I was rolled in a wheelchair through the United complex over to the Day Surgery Center early one morning where my wife was waiting for me. Up on the recovery room bed I went with my stylish hospital gown on for the stat checks, electrode placements, and the IV. The psychiatrist and anesthesiologist came in for each of their little talks, and the "all systems go" for the barrel roll maneuver. It was suggested that I make sure, for sure, to empty my bladder one last time in the nearby bathroom before the procedure because one effect of the induced seizure procedure is that it may cause me to "wet myself." When my turn came (they had three or four pre/post-op rooms), they rolled me into a simple room for the procedure: Psychiatrist to the left with his equipment, and Anesthetist under Anesthesiologist supervision on the right.

"Can you please state your name and birthdate?" I answer. "What procedure are you here for?" "Unilateral ECT," is my answer (they also do Bilateral ECT). I was snapped into all the electrodes, and all systems – a GO! Then the Anesthetist takes over stating, "Take deep breaths into the Ambu® bag. We give you a bit of something to numb, and then the anesthesia which may have a burning sensation for a second, and then you will be under in a couple seconds." Ready, set, barrel roll... yep, odd short burning sensation, and quick fuzziness as seen from my eyes, and I was out. From what I understand, they put a bite block in my mouth as this type of induced seizure causes a firm clenching of the jaw. The procedure does not last long. Back to the recovery room where, after the normal period of babbling and drooling for me, I slowly awakened and became conscious. Afterward, they checked my stats, gave me something to drink and snack on, and asked me if I felt well enough to leave. Then I was wheeled back to the cuckoo's nest, or driven home by Rita if it was an outpatient procedure.

Was my head spinning after the barrel roll maneuver? I felt a bit dizzy from the anesthesia, and basically tired for a while (if an outpatient procedure, you are not to drive or work the same day). I wet myself once. My jaw (TMJ joint) and cheek muscles were sore the rest of the day. My only suggestion, which I made being a former dentist, was for them to consider putting a TENS unit on the two joints as part of the post-op procedures while the patient is waking up, to help diminish the soreness and pain in the TMJ joints afterwards.

I do not use the word "miracle" lightly, but the procedure worked for me very well. Within a week (three treatments), I was not only released from the cuckoo's nest but feeling OK, as in, back to normal OK. I finished the 11th ECT treatment in May of 2019 and have been stable ever since. To be sure, making it through only 2 of the last 4 winters without a visit to the cuckoo's nest is not a trend yet, but I'll take it (writing this in February 2020). Yes, I am on a higher dose of Cymbalta than before, with a low dose of Seroquel at night in the winter, along with dutiful attention to eating, supplements, meditation, stretching/yoga, exercise, and light therapy. I know if I go down, and down hard and fast has been my MO, that I am doing all the "right things."

As odd as it might seem to a healthy person, I can honestly say I would rather have my brain shocked to the point of seizure than go through one more winter from hell with guesswork on medication changes, and a return visit to the cuckoo's nest. My psychiatrist and I have filed away ECT into my Emergency Flight Manual shall I need it again. When I have a mental health relapse, I seem to go into engine failure and a tail spin quickly. ECT pulled me quickly out of the crash and burn(out) stage of total despair and suicidal ideation.

> "Come to me, all you who labor and are heavily burdened, and I will give you rest. Take my yoke upon you and learn from me, for I am gentle and humble in heart; and you will find rest for your souls. For my yoke is easy, and my burden is light." Matthew 11:28-30

No Shortage of Other Flights
The Warriors – The Worn and Weary

Part of my journey in life is a spiritual one, and the spiritual tradition I grew up in and have studied follows the teaching of Jesus of Nazareth. Whether the divine spark within us is called the essence of self, heart of one's being, or one's soul, Mental Illness will challenge your perceptions severely when you enter a mental tailspin and abandonment of hope. In other words, it's a rift in your very being, your soul. I cannot tell you what the magic bullet, secret sauce, or rough-and-tumble answer is to recovery. I only have partial insights into my Mental Illness and health now after 30 years, and therefore am reticent to advise anyone else. But what I do know of anyone dealing with a Mental Illness is that they each are a warrior. I give credit for this insight to a member of one of the outpatient programs I participated in. When each of us were asked to describe ourselves or make a comment at the end of the program, the member stated, "I am a warrior."

In the quote from the gospel of Matthew attributed to Jesus of Nazareth listed above, I have found several truths about Mental Illness in the despair and hope, fear and tears, and life and death of those who suffer from some form of Mental Illness as I do. A battle is being waged by countless thousands each day with their own minds. It is not lost on me that a significant number lose that battle every year; several in my and my wife's family lost the battle through chronic self-medication of alcohol or from acute suicide by firearm. I and they are all warriors, but not of the triumph and glory type. These warriors are much more real and raw, a battle for life over death amidst their flight into Mental Illness, fought within one's own mind and also within an all too ignorant and unsympathetic battle waged but not always won. What I offer here is the following battlefield for MI warriors.

- Warrior by coming - searching and hoping
- Warrior by weariness - burden and hopelessness
- Warrior by openness - learning from otherness
- Warrior by yoke - tough work, can be lighter but always a yoke
- Warrior by yearning - much needed rest
- Warrior by self-love - gentleness and humility

Amidst the depression and/or anxiety there is a searching and hoping for answers within oneself. The why's, and the why me. Such a high flight into self-risk and fear leaves one gasping for oxygen to hold onto life itself. A battle - a warrior.

In the MI battle, with its tendency towards seclusion and/or avoidance, significant weariness and burden sets in. Everyone, and I mean everyone, has their limits of endurance of the mind. Bootstraps to pull oneself up by are in short supply, and sheer exhaustion sets in. Mix in self-doubt, fear, guilt, and potentially shame, and any person would find themselves in free fall of hopelessness. A battle - a warrior.

Now comes for some, including myself, the tough part. Yelling out to someone, anyone, for a parachute to allow for a rough but at least safe landing. It is the call or calls for help – the admission that you cannot help yourself any longer and to lay yourself upon the mercy and care of others. Life is at stake, and you learn to accept that you are not in your right mind. You are completely helpless, extremely vulnerable, and you stake your life on others and otherness. A battle - a warrior.

No joke, yoke it up instead. The effort needed is enormous to raise one's hopes in or for therapy, medication, exercise, meditation, etc.

while knowing that all of them will take a period of time to show any visceral signs of benefit. Pulling up with all your strength from a crash dive, not for some days but months in some cases, with no guarantee of success, is frankly a battle waged by a warrior.

Weakness does not drive a person in such a state, but the hope, although razor thin at times, for some needed rest. While guilt and shame plops one's mind into the swirling toilet of, "has it really come to this?", some semblance of rest is longed for when anything resembling normal is still out of sight and out of mind. A battle - a warrior.

It is not easy to love yourself enough to want to live or be humble enough to ask for help when you are not in your right mind or when society at large leads with a combination of ignorance, ridicule, and/ or avoidance. A battle – a warrior. Shhhh...best keep Mental Illness a secret in the shadows. Just pull yourself up by the bootstraps. Nothing can be that bad. Just believe in God, or worse, it's all in God's plan. I was blessed with an understanding and supportive wife, even amidst her justifiable questions, fear, and doubt (read her chapter). But many of these warriors face a battle not only with themselves, but within their families, and against an overwhelming societal force that wishes it to be ignored, ridiculed, or left in the shadows.

One irony for me is that illness, any illness, is basically a dis-ease of the self, but also the dis-ease caused for others is significant when the illness is brought into their reach and embrace. For this I am forever grateful, that while a lonely battle, I was not alone. I am convinced of one truism in this battle: that the outcome is more predictable when you have other unconditionally loving and courageous people by your side. The middle portion of the book is dedicated to them – those cherished few who walked through the locked doors of the cuckoo's nest to visit me.

SECTION TWO

Passengers Along on My Flight

Wife/Lifelong Partner – Rita

I am not a futuristic thinker/planner. I have never participated in doing a vision board type experience. (A vision board is any sort of board on which you display images that represent whatever you want to be, do, or have in your life.) On several occasions over my 61 years of life, I have been criticized for not "dreaming," "planning," or "putting it out there in the universe because then you are more likely to have it come true." I usually take things as they come and deal with it then. I remember back in the late 1990s, when Mick had the first "episode," and we talked about getting out of dentistry due to back pain. The first questions/concerns he had were… "What about the life you thought we would have together with me being a dentist and earning a certain income?" and "What about the type of house you thought we would be able to have?" and "What about the number of children you thought we would have?" My answer to him was… "I really never thought about those things!" Call me shallow, but maybe this has been beneficial for me as I travel the road of Mental Health with my husband, Mick.

I wish a vision board would come true and that I would have done one 37 years ago, when we got married, if this were the case. That vision board would NOT include several trips to the ER. It would NOT include experiencing the lock down unit at United Hospital that first time. It would NOT include watching my husband panicking, hyperventilating, and wondering what the hell is happening. It would NOT include wondering, at times, if Mick would be alive when I arrived home. And it would NOT include all the frustrations with both the medical and holistic communities as it relates to mental health. Over the past 37 years, I have been privileged to be married to a person who is a fighter and that is why this book is possible in 2020.

And now onto my perspective and experience regarding mental health from the past three years specifically. For me, I can categorize things into four areas - Emergency Rooms, Hospital Stays, Outpatient Treatments, and Daily Living/The New Normal.

I remember the first time experiencing the emergency room at United Hospital. We were escorted by police security personnel directly from the psychologist's office, through the many tunnels leading to United Hospital, into the ER admittance chair. That walk seemed VERY long with many eyes upon us and many heads averting our gaze as well. I had no idea what to expect (no vision board) but I wasn't surprised with how cold and scripted most employees were. Once admitted, Mick had to give up all his clothes and be dressed in scrubs. Additionally, we were put into a locked room with nothing on the walls where we waited for intake personnel to arrive. I remember asking (via an intercom) to go out to use the restroom. After the armed guard let me out, I glanced into the next locked room only to see a man writhing and screaming while lying on the floor in his own feces. Emergency room visits thereafter were frustrating, ugly, inhumane, and filled with long hours of waiting for a bed to become available.

The hospital stays were limited to two facilities: United Hospital and Hutchinson Hospital. The most memorable moment was after I left Mick the first time. I was trying to be strong for Mick and not show my emotions – my fear, my angst, my anger. When I was leaving, the man at the desk by the elevators saw my tears and he said, "Are you o.k.? Is this the first time here?" I sat and cried with him for a bit. He even came around from his desk to lay an empathetic hand on my shoulder. Little did I know that I would see him again after Mick was discharged, re-admitted to Hutchinson, and then returned again to United Hospital all within 4 months. When I did see him again, I thanked him for making a difference for me on that lonely night. The environments were so different between Hutchinson and United Hospitals and it opened my eyes to the inadequate ways "the system" deals with mental health in general. Facilities need to have windows, exercise equipment, single rooms, etc.

I have been a little more hopeful after experiencing the outpatient options as Mick and I traveled this journey. The psychologists, psychiatrists, and other professionals who ran the partial hospitalization program and the day treatment programs were supportive, responsive to our needs, and shared the frustration with how we treat the mental health needs that are increasing. The other outpatient treatment Mick received was Electroconvulsive Therapy (ECT) and again, I came away hopeful, though it was very hard to see my husband looking and feeling basically "o.k." and then coming out of the treatment so tired and "out of it" for a period of time.

Many times it propelled my thinking into the future and what it might look like when we will need to take care of each other because of other medical conditions perhaps (still not going to do a vision board!). The "new normal" and daily living has changed forever especially after Mick had another "episode" last year. I better understand that this is a disease and not something that Mick, nor anyone for that matter, can just "pull themselves up by the bootstraps" and stop. I have learned that doing "self-care" is way different than being selfish, although it might appear one is being selfish. I am less tolerant of people who criticize the use of medication as a means to help someone who is depressed and anxious. I am also irritated by people who preach that just one approach will "make it better" - i.e. aromatherapy, meditation, yoga, etc. I am more knowledgeable about mental health issues in general as I have read a lot and have participated in resources offered through the National Alliance on Mental Illness (NAMI). More importantly, I have lived with someone who suffers from this disease, in big and small ways, for 37 years. I have learned that I need to take care of myself and that I am not responsible for Mick's Mental Health – only he can decide how he will manage this disease and I will help in ways that I can. This is why I continue to be engaged with my family and friends even when Mick cannot. This is why we have open/honest conversations. This is why I seek out my own therapist and my own self-care.

And now for MY personal version of a Vision Board moving forward as it relates to Mental Illness.

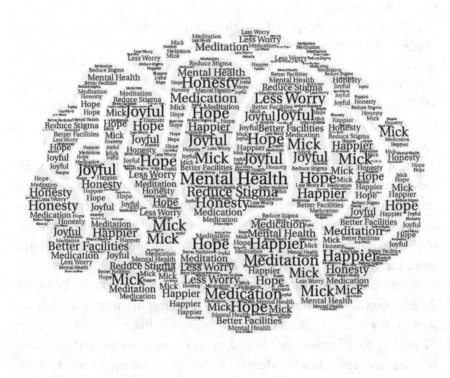

Daughter – Teresa

I become increasingly aware, through my personal experience and those of others, how delicate yet powerful our minds are. We are intrinsically connected to one another, whether we are conscious of it or not in each moment, despite living in a culture that encourages us to be self-serving or self-sufficient. Connection is delightful in times of joy and celebration, but painful in times of suffering.

My father's journey with anxiety and depression is uniquely his but also shared and transferred into the fabric of my lived experience and all those others you hear from in this collection. I could recount the past four years chronologically; to reflect on each onset date, inpatient hospitalization, changes in drug regimens, or the treatments outside the hospital he received. However, this could create the perception that we've 'gotten through' a period in our shared experience as a family, that I've gathered the data I need to personally reconcile the painful experiences of seeing him suffer, or that in the absence of severe symptoms or lapses that each of our mental health doesn't still warrant special attention and care.

The continuum of personal mental health can change day to day and moment to moment, even in the absence of a diagnosable condition. This was not an existing awareness I had, but one that confronted me head on after I welcomed my first child and experienced the alarming shift in energy expenditure and self-care away from myself onto another human being through pregnancy, childbirth, and nursing. My maternity leave was October through January, some of our darker days in Minnesota where hibernation occurs for not only animals but people also. There were great times of joy, but also loneliness. My assumption that this would dissolve as I returned to work and he got older was met with disappointment as those feelings crept back in through his development at various times. I didn't "defeat" it.

I would say that to some degree, but less, this returned with my second child. Baby boy number two was 'on board' during my father's second round of hospitalizations as an inpatient. During our visits, my dad started talking more openly about some of the treatment approaches he was engaging in, including Cognitive Behavioral Therapy (CBT). A hallmark of CBT is the recognition of the interaction between our thoughts, behaviors, and emotions related to the homeostasis of our mental well-being. It resonated for whatever reason. The idea that all thoughts and emotions are just that, thoughts and emotions and warrant our attention but maybe not a reactive behavior. A light illuminated you could say, the changes I experienced after my first pregnancy in regards to my mental health required my attention.

Mild social anxiety surfaced about 6-8 months after giving birth to my second child who was in utero during those visits to my Dad. Due to physical body changes, the overwhelming mental load of trying to locate and ensure the safety of my eldest while nursing my second, and simultaneously trying to carry on a meaningful conversation with a neighbor was suffocating. But this time, it was suffocating enough that it was changing my behavior. It took me awhile to recognize my irritability with my spouse, my avoidance of social engagements, or how the negative thoughts of unworthiness were limiting my ability to seek help and health. This was the crossroads for me; whether it was a moment, or a day, or a period of time, I cannot recall. I decided seeking an evaluation with a therapist was the best decision. To share that it took me nearly two and a half years to come to that moment of action, another seven months before I told another soul outside my family that I was attending therapy, and another six months to phase out of therapy – I hope it encourages any eyes that read.

I have not arrived at a conclusion that most final paragraphs should contain. Settling into the expectation that my Mental Health, in addition to my father's, will continue to be fluid and ever evolving is not comfortable or easy. However, it has given me a sense of permission or forgiveness for when some of my unwelcomed metaphorical guests – stress, sadness, shame, or loneliness – return. Rumi, mentions in his poem, "The Guest House" (2004), that every morning is a new arrival. That we should try to welcome any and every metaphorical guest...they may be clearing you out for a new delight. My hope for myself, my father, and anyone else is to move towards enjoyment of these "new delights." For now... in this moment... for me, it is the increased dedication I have to care for and not be scared by my delicate and powerful mind.

Daughter - Katie

The Daughter that Lived Away

Through my dad's recent episodes of worsening or change in Mental Illness, including his in-patient hospital stays and outpatient programs, I did not live near my parents. I was a plane ride or two away, living in Michigan and New Hampshire. My experience was very different from that of my sister's, Mom's, and even my dad's close friends, because I didn't see and hear the day-to-day. I think everyone has had some sort of experience where it's "if you weren't there, then you just don't know." Certainly, it was true in this case for me. I didn't, and still don't truly know or fully understand everything that went on during those months. What I do remember is talking to my dad on the phone and him saying tearfully "I don't know if I am going to see you again." I think my next words simultaneously to my mom (on the phone) and husband (next to me) were "What is going on?!" I knew my dad was anxious, depressed, not feeling well, medications were not working, etc... But I didn't know it was "that bad" or "to that point."

Thankfully, I was able to visit on occasion and those visits were essential for me to support my dad, my mom, my sister and to process the episodes, Mental Health system, and my own feelings. On a few occasions, I packed up my daughter Emelia who was an infant at the time, put her in the baby carrier, and off I went to the airport. My family has had really raw open conversations and learned a lot through these experiences. We have learned how to better support my dad and each other. We have learned through trial and error what to say and what not to say. We have learned that it's okay to ask directly and specifically how someone is doing instead of "how are things" which elicits the typical response, "fine." We have learned that when my dad says "I need to go for a walk", "I need a break", or "I need to leave" it is not him being antisocial or rude. It is him taking care of himself and responding to his environment and establishing boundaries.

A few things surprised me (negatively and positively) about the awareness and acceptance of mental health during these past four years. First was, my job did not approve my days off request to visit my dad. Yes, my supervisor knew the reason and severity. I didn't fight it, I instead called in sick for the days I needed. Second, was that many well-meaning people days or weeks after the in-hospital stays would ask "So everything is good now, right?!" or "Oh good he's out of the hospital, are you relieved?" The wording or how it was said didn't sit right with me because Mental Illness is a lifelong illness. While episodes may subside or medications may make someone more stable— no everything is not "good." No, my dad wasn't "all better." Yes, I was relieved in a sense that he was discharged from the hospital, but it's not like other illnesses or hospitalizations where a discharge means it is all done/over. It was hard to respond because I knew my response was not what they were hoping to hear. Third, is the gap in services and programs for mental health. Psychiatrists and psychologists can take months to get into even if you are an established patient. You can't get into outpatient programs without seeing a doctor first and getting referred. And the only thing left when things are bad enough or urgent enough is to go to the ER. To sit in one of the most anxiety inducing and depressing places I can think of and wait. Fourth, is that there are support groups for families through NAMI and other local organizations. It may take a bit to find them, but they are there. And lastly, the more my family and I shared the more we heard similar stories of "you aren't alone" and found the people we could rely on, to talk to, to just sit with.

On a personal note, I have a history of anxiety and depression dating back to my middle school years surrounding friendships, then focusing in high school, test anxiety, and feeling sad for "no clear reason." It has always been part of my life in bigger or smaller ways. While my dad was going through his journey in and out of the "cuckoo's nest," I was also transitioning to being a brand-new mom, living away from family with a husband working long hours, finding a new "tribe" of friends, and adjusting to a new job. I have moved two more times since then, more job changes for myself and husband, another daughter added to our family, amongst many other things. Lots of change and stress layered on possible postpartum anxiety and/or depression. I have come to have more acceptance that anxiety and depression is part of my story and does not define me.

So, I think what I take away from all of this is if I struggle with anxiety and depression: to share, be open, be honest, be vulnerable, and seek help. I personally am going to try to be an established patient that is connected with a psychologist because you just never know when life situations and stress become too much to handle. And you certainly can't predict when an episode of worsening anxiety or depression will happen. Getting a Mental Health check-up should be as routine or more routine than getting your physical check-up with a doctor. While sharing about a physical ailment seems very easy, there is hesitation around people sharing about how they are doing mentally. The "invisible illnesses" are the hardest to understand. So I suggest the following to someone attending to someone who may be struggling mentally: to listen, ask questions, don't assume, be present, and be open. And on both ends of the Mental Health experience, may we advocate to reduce the stigma around Mental Illness and advocate for more/better mental health services so my dad, myself, and everyone else can more easily access the services they need.

Mother - Lorraine

My knowledge of depression illness was very minimal, but by asking questions, I learned a great deal. I had always hoped that as parents we would never get a phone call informing us that one of the children had been admitted to a Mental Hospital. I did, however, receive a phone call informing me that you were admitted to a Mental Health Unit in St. Paul. My first reaction was to cry and then I picked up my rosary beads and started to pray that you were fine. My Faith has been my stronghold for my journey along the road in good times and bad. My emotions at this point were pretty high. After a day or two, I had the opportunity to visit you and found that you were doing well and, with the help of the psychiatrist and staff, you would be discharged in a week or two.

You have made a few more trips to the Mental Health Unit in St. Paul but when you needed to be admitted again the hospitals in the Twin Cities were occupied so you were admitted to the one in Hutchinson. When we (wife Rita and niece Mel, and I) went to visit you there, we found it more spacious with private rooms for each patient. When we visited you there, we played the card game "Salad." Had lots of fun but I do not know who won – I assume it was you or Melanie. I knew when we left that day you would soon be discharged.

While there, during leisure time, you pencil colored pictures printed in a book. I do not know how many you colored but I was the recipient of one that was a heart-shaped fishbowl, colored to perfection. It is a reminder to me of you and Dad and your love of fishing at Sparkling Lake in Canada. I will treasure it forever. I love you, Mick.

Friend - Gordy

I'm old enough to worry—in fact, I'm *very* experienced at it as well. So, I will begin my chapter by confessing to "feeling anxious" as I begin to write it. You see, I have kept a detailed journal of my life, for *every* day of it, since January 1st of 1970. So, before I began writing my chapter about Mick and Mental Health—or Illness—I looked into my journal for my account of the day that I went to visit Mick on the Mental Health Floor at United Hospital in St. Paul. And there was no account of it! Search as I have, I simply could not find any written summary of my visit to Mick that surreal day that I went to visit him. That is very, very uncharacteristic of me, that I would have failed to enter a summary of our visit on that day.

And that worries me, because it forces me to ask myself if I should be worried that I might be starting to lose my memory. And then my worry ratchets up to anxiety, because I realize I can no longer remember names and phone numbers and events and dates as infallibly as I once did. And then it hits me: this is such "small potatoes" compared to what Mick has been dealing with for years—and I am humbled, and even a bit ashamed by how true this is. But, for what it's worth, it reinforces for me the truth that there are many, many levels and degrees and kinds of Mental Illness—and beyond our worries about our own trivial memory lapses, there are terrifying varieties of Mental Illness that society simply chooses to ignore or—worse still—simply pretends they're not there.

And then a special friend like Mick comes along, and he is so open about his Mental Illness issues that his humble honesty and forthrightness simply lower your socially engendered typical "buffer zones" against such an "unmentionable" illness and lets you dare look into it, to come to better understand and more truthfully acknowledge it. As Pogo so eloquently said years ago, "We have seen the enemy, and it is us." Until we acknowledge the existence of Mental Illness and address society's veiled ignorance and denial of it, we cannot manage, treat, and lessen the effects of Mental Illness and disorders that have been with us since we first became erect and began using our brains.

I give Mick credit for inspiring me to address my own inability and fear to acknowledge the reality of Mental Illness: here at last was a dear friend who openly talked about his own Mental Illness—and taught me that it plays no favorites and spares no classes in whom it affects.

Because of Mick, I could finally put my ignoring of Mental Illness into a resolvable question: Why do people not question the fact that people can have "heart" disease (I have it) or "pancreatic" disease (diabetes—I have that, too!) or cancer or Parkinson's Disease or MS, but *do* question that people can have "brain" disease? Of all the major organs in the body, why would the brain be the only one not subject to illness, to disease? Why should the brain be given such exclusivity, granted such immunity from disease? The answer is, it shouldn't and it can't be, and to ignore this truth—perhaps because it manifests itself in behaviors more disturbing and unsettling to others than the diseases of the other organs do—is to extend to people who are honestly ill a grave and unconscionable disservice.

So, still being unable to find the exact dates and entries for my interactions with Mick during his "encounters" with ANDY, I will— God help us all—have to rely on my memory as I continue here.

Where I get a bit mixed up is in what happened during which session of institutionalization—but, since my imperfect memory cannot pinpoint the exact time for these episodes, it raises the question of how important correct sequential order is. So that I can continue with my narration, I am ruling that it is not that important to what I am going to share.

(And, before I go any further, I would like to call attention to that big, long word in the preceding paragraph: *institutionalization*. Doesn't that word scare the sh—oops—send chills up and down your spine? What a *horrible* word! Just what, exactly, **is** an *institution*? It certainly doesn't sound very home-y and warm, does it? It sounds rather cold and impersonal and unyielding and overly regimented to me, and it conjures in my mind old-movie images of imposing, stolid, massive, castle-like structures built of huge blocks punctuated by barred windows, with lightning flashing and thunder pealing and wind-driven rain pelting against it. And so, just in thinking of my dear friend Mick being institutionalized, my soul was filled with horror and dread.)

Okay: I remember a very somber call from Rita in late fall or early winter, telling me that Mick had lapsed into another bout with ANDY, and that the only place with a bed for Mick was way out in Hutchinson. It took me a day or two to ratchet up my courage to decide that I was going to Hutchinson to visit Mick—and then I got another call from Rita saying that Mick had now been moved to United Hospital, as a bed had opened up there for him, a bed much nearer to Hastings than Hutchinson. (And, as relieved as I was to hear that, I must admit, I never did find out if the facility in Hutchinson really was as impregnable-castle-like as I had imagined.)

With Mick now in an in-town hospital, I called Rita and coordinated with her what would be the best time for me to visit Mick in the Mental Health Ward at United Hospital, and so it was that I went to United to visit Mick on a weekday afternoon.

And I *was* nervous about the visit, because I had never before visited someone hospitalized in the Mental Health Ward. True to my nature, my biggest concern was that I "say all the right things" to Mick—in other words, nothing that might upset or disturb him. Because I am in the habit of always saying a prayer to the Holy Spirit before engaging in a conversation that likely will be emotional, uncomfortable, confrontational, or otherwise challenging, I did just that, asking for composure and naturalness and the grace for my love and concern for him to shine through whatever I said to him, or however I reacted to him.

But all this normal mental and emotional focus and calming was soon blown away as I exited the elevator and proceeded to a locked door equipped with a camera and intercom. I pressed the button and was greeted by an inquiry of whom I was here to see, and then I was buzzed through that first set of doors and confronted by a wall of lockers and a set of printed instructions for what I must do before entering through the second set of doors, also equipped with a camera and intercom. I was directed to leave my watch, wallet, and keys in a locker, *along with my pants belt and shoelaces.* It was only then that it hit me, that in visiting Mick I must bring no items in with me with which he might be able to harm (or worse) himself—or might be snatched from me by another patient, for similar use. I suddenly realized this visiting people in a Mental Health Ward is very, very serious business, and it grieved me to think that my kind, generous, compassionate friend Mick was literally being kept in so almost dehumanizing an environment. So, finally "pared" down to the required clothing specifications, I buzzed at the second door and was admitted into the Mental Health Ward.

And there was Mick, leaning over a table, working on a complex coloring-for-adults picture, and a lot of my disorientation disappeared in seeing him look up and recognizing me. He stood up to greet me with a faint smile and look of utter gratitude, and it was the Ol' Mick himself, welcoming and as caring as ever. Yes, he looked a bit muted and wan—perhaps even a bit washed-out—but, after all, who wouldn't be, after all the upheaval and exams and evaluations and trials with new medication combinations? He spoke slowly and deliberately, and, while, in being faithful to my confession of mild forgetfulness, I must say I cannot recall all of what we talked about, I do remember how wonderful it was to be conversing with him, and realizing that the resilient inner core of who Mick is had surmounted all trials and issues and was still working on all levels, even if somewhat muted: personal, spiritual, and psychological. What I *do* remember with crystal clarity is that he seemed somewhat distracted and would often look expectantly over my shoulder, to the extent that at some point, he felt obligated to tell me that he was awaiting his psychiatrist and was feeling fairly confident that he was being discharged today. I could see both hope and joy growing within him, and suddenly he saw the doctor come in and excused himself, eager to hear what his psychiatrist had to say. I fully understood his immediate engagement with his doctor, and so I got up, wished him good luck and a discharge today, and said goodbye to him.

As I emerged from the Ward and then the changing room, and walked down a sunlit hall to the elevator, I felt myself filled with joy and hope for Mick, and I said a silent prayer that his wish would be granted, that he would be able to go home to his family that day. I later learned that he did.

I must say, the Mental Health Ward at United did not seem like part of the everyday world, and I am sure that by its very nature whoever is hospitalized there feels, to some degree, disoriented and flawed and segregated and forgotten and hidden away, out of shame. And all that is wrong, it seems to me. For the past nine years, I have been bringing Communion to the patients of St. Joseph Hospital in St. Paul, and in all my entries and exits from rooms in the ICU and post-surgery unit, I never experienced any patient feeling shame for whatever condition brought him or her to the hospital. We all understood that illness is a part of the human condition, and that one goes to a hospital to be healed, to find recovery.

But there is that stigma to Mental Illness that refuses to go away, which is so unfair: again, brains and their chemistry can "become ill" every bit as naturally as hearts and livers and kidneys and bones, but, for those with Mental Illness, shame is too often part of that package. One must know someone who lives with Mental Illness in order to come to realize that while they are fighting the disease, they are *still* people, *still* the dear friend or family member, or kind, gentle soul we have always known them to be. And we must walk with them in support and acceptance and patience and love. As I think back on my visit with Mick that day, the analogy that comes to my mind is that I walked into a dark place with fear but with a candle held high to help me find my beloved friend, and that, when the light of my candle (the love I have in my heart for him) illuminated his face, he experienced the joy of knowing that he was loved and valued and welcomed back to a world of normalcy and light and purpose.

Two final thoughts to tack on here: 1) I am proud to tell you that my daughter Laura chose to major in Psychology and earn a Master's Degree in Counseling, to work with people with Mental Illness and its accompanying shame and lack of confidence—she has always had so kind and loving and caring a heart, and it is inspiring to me to see her choosing to spend her life helping those living with Mental Illness, at an income level that does not at all reflect the importance to society of the work she does; and 2) in knowing that Mick's healing treatment led him to Electroshock Therapy, I am reminded of my Mother's dear cousin and friend Johanna, who spent several years at the St. Peter's Hospital in St. Peter, the first hospital specializing in the treatment of the mentally ill in the state, sometime during the late 1940s or early 1950s. Johanna was what some would call "a poor soul," in that she was shy and quiet and withdrawn—and always picked on by her older sisters and scolded by her mother. And so, it was only natural that my Mother would befriend her and invite her to every one of our family functions and gatherings, always treating her with kindness and unconditional love and deep respect—and empathy. She once told me that Johanna had shared with her that she had undergone extensive shock therapy while at St. Peter—and it made me glad that a treatment viewed so darkly by most people in that earlier era would survive in the world of psychiatry through all those years and be "tweaked" to the extent that it is now an approved treatment for depression and some other mental disorders. For me, it forged a bridge between Johanna and Mick that stretched over a long span of years, based on a shared mental disease—and it brought me a sense of encouragement that, with its modern acceptability in the medical world, *perhaps* we are making progress in our approach to and treatment of Mental Illnesses.

I would like to end with some brazen plagiarism—of my own words from a memory I shared with Mick in his surprise retirement book—and it's about this use of electric current to treat areas of the brain:

> *Still, my dearest memory of time spent with you [Mick] is on a road trip of another sort, when you caught a ride up to St. Paul for your final Electroshock Therapy at United Hospital, and needed a ride back home afterward. As I pulled into the circular drive to pick you up, you walked out to my car in a daze and slumped into the passenger seat of my car. Our conversation was very limited that day, as we spoke in short sentences and partial phrases—obviously electroshock treatments are no picnic. As I watched you almost sleepwalk to the door of your house, my heart was awash with love and compassion for you—along with a sincere prayer for healing sleep for you. It hit me wordlessly, all the trusting love you have for me as a friend, to honor me by*

> *letting me see you and help you in your utmost vulnerability,*
> *in the nakedness of the gaping swath of emotional and physical*
> *damage that depression can wreak in so pure and beautiful and*
> *innocent a soul as yours. To be able to bring your dear friend*
> *home to healing and rest and recovery—what greater grace than*
> *that can there be?*

When something so devastating can happen to so dear a friend as Mick, it reminds us that it can and does happen to others and even ourselves. It is such friends as Mick who teach us of the horrors of Mental Illness, and society's moral obligation to recast it in a proper light, as a disease that can hide and swallow-up the person in whom it takes quarter, and a disease that cries for more research and funding and greater availability to all—so that we can more effectively limit the damage to the individual and society as a whole. When all is said and done, Mental Illness is indeed a disease as deserving of healing as any other bodily illness.

When we bring the love of Christ for those living with Mental Illness into our hearts and then bring his desire for their healing to society, perhaps then we can change the equation on Mick's ANDY to ring true for all, "And He walks with me, and He talks with me. And He tells me I am His own. And the joy we share as we tarry there, none other has ever known."

Amen.

Friend – Peter

Anyone who grew up in the upper Midwest knows that fall (at least in my opinion) is the most beautiful of the seasons. Warm days, cool nights, and a break from the summer heat and humidity and time to begin slowing down before the onslaught of winter. Still, the most beautiful of fall days can so quickly turn into what we know is coming – winter – and suddenly it is upon us. As one who grew up in North Dakota and has spent the last 40 years in Minnesota, I took pride in thinking I'm ready, "bring it on." How foolish and naïve I was!

Muffler Grouping (we thought we could change our own mufflers on our own cars ourselves) became the safe way to grow our friendship. This was a manly way to get to know this new friend. How much damage could we do, it's only a muffler? We met through a church retreat just for men, and quickly began sharing first our blessings and all the facets of our lives that were safe to tell others about. You see, you don't want to scare people away, especially new friends, by revealing too much, especially the truth. But in time, a rather short time, the more intensely, truly dark moments in our respective lives, the loss of life, and the loss of purpose were shared. Soon we were helping to carry one another. Nothing heroic, nothing particularly noteworthy, except for periodic episodes of two guys sitting in the front seats of a Ford Escort or Toyota Corolla (both with pretty good exhaust systems), and sobbing in the parking lot while holding hands and occasionally offering a hug over the stick shift.

"Would you like to go fishing to Sparkling Lake, Canada, with my Dad and a few other guys?" Was there any possible answer except "Yes, if it is okay with Kath." On that first trip, as we are sitting in the canoe, as he looks at my face and says, "Oh, that was the biggest fish you've ever caught?" as he throws it back. "Don't worry, that is just a hammer handle, there will be more, and they will be keepers." And then for another trip there was, "Oh, it is only 5 portages to 'Kasishy,'" and waking up to Mel working on breakfast when we had made it there, while Mick and Pat were taking a 6 am bath. I was thinking "this is nuts," but I strip down and damn near kill myself falling into the lake. Then, there was the one word shouted over the roar of a 15-hp motor on the way to the north end of Sparkling for evening fishing as dark, ugly rain clouds were rolling in, after I informed Mick that I had forgotten my rain gear back in camp. "Bummer," he said. It forever holds the greatest lesson I have ever learned at Sparkling; I have never again forgotten my raingear!

Yes, there have been other memories, such as chasing elk outside Estes Park, CO. Trips to Red Lake with students and family were memorable as well. While doing bicycle ride-support through Iowa with Mick, reenacting a pivotal scene from *Field of Dreams* with Anne in Dyersville, pork chops that looked more like T-bone steaks, and a 4th of July in McGregor that was straight out of a Rockwell painting, were all memorable too.

I thought I knew him, and I thought we'd faced our darkest moments 30 years prior, and by the grace of God and the gift of friendship, we had overcome them together. "Does anyone know where the love of God goes when the waves turn the minutes to hours?" I thought, pridefully and naively, that I was ready for whatever may come next. The girls go out to get their nails done, which I think was just code for "I need someone to talk to, to listen. I need a break!" I'm working on supper, and you are curled up in the fetal position on the couch and you say to me in a voice of utter exhaustion, "I know you've got a gun in the house, and you'd be doing me a favor!"

"Does anyone know where the love of God goes when the waves turn the minutes to hours?" There I was, knowing that I will forever be looking in from the outside. Each minute, each breath, each thought, a darkness and despair that I hope to never know. Yes, losing Teresa, my first daughter shortly after birth was a darkness, and emptiness that I pray others will never be confronted with. Yes, it was a loss that took years to recover from, but there was some finality, some semblance of closure. But there you are on my couch, then at United Hospital, also Hutchinson, and "it" is inside of you. I've come to realize, and I know I'll never fully appreciate that this "it" can't be buried in a cemetery with a marker to remind others what was lost. Instead, this "it" must be dug up, confronted, exposed for what it is, Mental Illness. You don't get a marker.

Because of your love of your family, and by the grace of God, you know that this is bigger than you and in great humility you reach out and accept the help that many others run from or are shamed into not accessing. Even as the darkness overcomes you, you are so gracious, so generous with your expressions of gratitude to all who provide care. Still, I said to him, "Mick, this is like a cancer, this is bad eyesight, this is a broken bone. You didn't do something reckless to bring this upon yourself. You are loved and so very loveable and deserve to be happy, to be well." You are so gentle with others in their woundedness, and over time, permit yourself to be gentle to yourself.

While I believed in my heart all that I was saying, a feeling of helplessness was often being hidden, suppressed. My short visits were so little compared to the hours and hours of work that were required of you for weeks on end. I had fear over saying the wrong thing, offering a poorly-assumed comparison, wondered whether humor was appropriate, and were questions about therapy, group, and medications, or Rita helpful? My minutes…Your hours. Where was the love of God?

Years earlier, when our families would come together for meals, you would offer a prayer that wasn't "Bless us oh Lord, and these thy gifts…" Instead, *"I believe in the sun even when it is not shining, I believe in love even when I cannot feel it, I believe in God even when God is silent."*

I'm not one filled with great insight or wisdom. I do believe with all my heart in a God who loves us, who believes in us, and in that belief hopes that we choose what is good and right and holy. In other words, we have free will. Readers, forgive my bluntness, but "shit happens." "It" happens not by the hand of God to test or punish us, but because sometimes we've made bad choices, sometimes because someone else made a bad choice that impacts us, and sometimes "it" happens just because. Life can be messy and hard, really, really hard at times because of that messiness. And life can be really, really good. As you so often alluded to, even in some of your most difficult times, that one need only look around with eyes of gratitude to see the goodness, blessings, and beauty that surrounds us.

It was a privilege to be there, to be trusted by you and Rita. To be a companion with you on this particular leg of your journey has been a blessing. As I encounter students who have dug holes that for all practical purposes will be impossible to climb out of, I ask myself, what are they bringing with them today that few, if anyone, knows about, including me? What is their story that they've learned to "live with," even accepted as normal? Your trust, your permitting me to sit at your side, your willingness to reveal your darkness, though at times scaring the hell out of me and sometimes prompting me to want to run from it, has made me a better person. Thank you.

You ask about my impressions of the Mental Health system, and my thoughts and insights are limited. Each day at school, I am profoundly grateful for my colleagues in the Counseling Office with whom I share a space. Daily, a steady stream of kids, some because they have to, but many because they want to, recognizing their need for some support, reach out for help. Life is messy, especially for our adolescents and young adults. The lack of trust in one or several, such as, government, law enforcement, politicians, religious leaders, all contribute to what can feel like a very bleak world. As never before, the need for support with maintaining one's mental health, especially for our young people, is profound. With that said, I see more and more of my students who are encumbered by the diagnosis of "clinically depressed" or experiencing Mental Illness. There is an increasingly healthy attitude of "I don't care, I'm not afraid of the label."

"I believe in the sun even when it is not shining, I believe in love even when I cannot feel it, I believe in God even when God is silent"

Thank you, my friend for not just speaking, but faithfully living the profound truth held in that prayer.

SECTION THREE

The Touch Down Affection for the Afflicted - Why Keep Flying

Empathy nudges one to shut up and listen,
sympathy prods one to come up with something
clever while planning one's escape

The Reaction
"You are No Good to Us Dead"

Later in this portion of the book, I will land upon some of what I have and have not found can be helpful in dealing with Mental Illness. For now, I wish to take off on the subject of what others, from family members and co-workers to mental health systems, can do or say that impacts one's flight in or toward the cuckoo's nest. While an oversimplification, it boils down to a choice: become more aware and knowledgeable, or simply avoid, ignore, or even be dismissive and cruel toward Mental Illness.

Case in point is the quote at the top under the title. During my first flight into the cuckoo's nest straddling 2016/2017, I was struggling not only with starting back to work or not, but also with adding to my transparency with my two bosses and HR in needing additional time off for the partial inpatient program. It crossed my mind whether I would lose my job as a chaplain; I was nervous as I approached them. Both of my bosses were empathetic, one sharing knowledge of such a crisis having personally gone through hospitalization as a teenager. Then I approached HR from which the above quote comes from. After explaining that I had talked with both bosses, and would need more time away to attend to my mental health and recovery, he stated his understanding and then, "You are no good to us dead." I was suffering and struggling to stay alive, as in white knuckles hanging onto life struggling, and the HR person just threw a verbal bomb into my brain's crash dive. Ignorant, insensitive son-of-a-bitch I thought to myself as I departed. Then I remembered what my first therapist said to me 30 years ago, "Mick, if you only had an eyeball hanging out of its socket, people might understand."

Awareness leads to understanding, and understanding leads to a choice, a fork in the road; either you become more empathetic towards another or you choose to avoid and/or deny the situation (subject of the next chapter). I wish to share a couple other quotes here before launching into the reaction of true empathy.

While useful, I am not talking merely about being aware of insensitive language. Where I worked, Corporate started a Mental Illness awareness initiative called "Be the Change." Discouraging use of ignorant colloquialisms was the crux of the initiative from my observation. Be careful not to say phrases such as, "I'm having a crazy day," "that's just nuts," or "are you insane!" was the motto. This from the same organization that had the small, dimly lit, noisy inpatient unit I stayed in twice.

Perhaps a bit brutal, but I thought of it as merely institutional fluff. It seemed a way for an organization that knows mental health is a huge issue to claim it is doing something by making a minimalistic investment. It looked good on the comprehensiveness and continuum of care charts and stats they are so fond of showing. After I had recovered from my fourth inpatient stay in that Twin Cities facility that also ran the hospital where I worked in my hometown as chaplain, the corporate CEO sent out a typical monthly message. This time the CEO had a closer encounter with Mental Illness from someone she knew and was trying to be sympathetic toward the seriousness of Mental Illness. After I read the message, I emailed the CEO and stated basically that if a firsthand opinion and knowledge from an employee who experienced the spectrum of the company's current mental health services would prove helpful, I would be glad to sit down for a chat. I never got a response.

I will not bore you with statistics, as I did in another book, as you can look up the personal and social cost of Mental Illness in terms of life, money, and relationships by looking up organizations such as National Alliance on Mental Illness (NAMI) or World Health Organization (WHO). I will simply say, from myself and you, from families to churches, from communities to healthcare systems, to society itself, we all must change our awareness and knowledge, and hopefully empathy, toward Mental Illness. Why is it that the "sky has no limits" in research, in personnel, and in money for bowels and bladders, beating hearts, breathing, and breasts, but not for the brain that runs them all? Why is it that the cause of Mental Illness can barely take off when it is one of the costliest health issues of our or any time? A shortage of beds and Mental Health professionals of all kinds at this point is what – brainless?! I feel that the engrained reaction to Mental Illness needs to change; lives are at stake, family relations are at stake, and even if you are a zero-sum game type, significant economic strain on society is at stake.

The Recognition
Only the Shadow Knows

There is a double-edged sword within the quotes above for me. The more mentally healthy part of me totally agrees with being "enlightened" by the "darkness," but when I relapse the most, I wouldn't wish Andy on my worst enemy's enemy. As I delved into the "darkness" earlier in the book, I will focus on the potential of enlightenment here. It does no one any good for Andy to be left in the shadows – not the person suffering, not loved ones, not mental health professionals trying to assist, nor society at large. But my opinion is that hiding Mental Illness from recognition, discussion, and acceptance is exactly where the bulk of society is; it is best mentioned in a quiet hushed tone, if at all.

As a Deacon in the Catholic tradition, I offer my services to a retreat program. In a leadership meeting with about 12 participants one evening in December 2019, the warm-up question for all to consider was on the lines of, "when was a time that you were emotionally drained or in distress, and who or what was of assistance in that journey?" As I have told limited parts of my story opening in public homilies in church, and more extensively when appropriate in the retreat program, I took the lead and mentioned my four recent visits in the last three years to a cuckoo's nest. Besides the professional help, I mentioned the assistance provided to me by the limited number (contributors in this book) of individuals who were willing to walk through those locked doors and visit with me.

My openness in front of this leadership group, who knew and loved me as a Christian brother, drew others to share their own personal or close encounters with Mental Illness. All but two of those twelve present had significant encounters with Mental Illness within their own family or they had suffered from it themselves. No extensive double-blind study here of course, but I severely doubt that the open sharing would have taken place if I had not shared the raw presence of Andy in my life first. I also have no doubt that such sharing or open dialogue rarely, if ever, occurs amongst casual friends or within most families.

Andy remains in the shadows for a number of reasons, probably only a partial list would include personal, familial, and societal factors. The person dealing with Andy suffers from confusion, frustration, anger, guilt, and potentially shame over it. Many family members don't know how to respond and/or deny its existence. Finally, society does not look kindly on those who are mentally ill; from shaming to blaming to ignoring, society is generally unkind and/or unempathetic to those dealing with Mental Illness.

From my Christian scripture tradition, I see those Jesus of Nazareth approached who were "demon possessed," shouting uncontrollably, and/or frothing at the mouth, as the population of his time who were suffering from Andy to one extent or another. In Jesus' time, they were considered unclean and were some of the untouchables, numbered amongst the outcasts not to be spoken to. While softened a bit in our time, in many ways nothing has changed. I believe society generally, as I did as well initially, thinks that Mental Illness is a flaw or weakness in the person. That thinking is a cruel form of judgment.

When I worked at Hastings Family Service many years ago, and during my relatively stable 15-20 years with Andy, I could not imagine getting so bad I would need to be checked into a cuckoo's nest. I remember one individual that approached us at HFS on behalf of a relative due to that relative's emotional instability and inability to care for themselves. One late afternoon that relative all but carried his disturbed relative into the back seat of a minivan to drive him up to the Cities to check the relative into a cuckoo's nest. I thought with less than empathy, "Wow, that person is really messed up!"

Any Mental Illness shadow is difficult to define, as typically a number of factors are involved: genetic/familial disposition, general health, level of diet and exercise, stress factors of all sorts, and level of connection with otherness (family, friends, spiritual). I have only a partial, but growing grasp, of the complexity of those factors within my life, and as stated earlier, I am reluctant to describe another's Andy shadow. That said, I firmly believe, to the core of my being, that all that I am must be attentive to Andy if I am going to remain mentally stable. What motivates me in this regard, is part wisdom and part fear.

As an apples and oranges analogy perhaps, I get together occasionally with a recent work friend of mine who suffers from alcoholism and has been sober for 20+ years. When a few acquaintances ask him, "With your long sobriety, perhaps you can successfully go back to light social drinking." He just shook his head when he told me this and said, "Why would I take that chance; why would I risk it? All I know is what has worked: going to AA meetings, and staying away from old haunts and certain tempting circumstances."

That is how I currently feel about my Mental Health. I do what works for me: watching my diet (aka - garbage in leads to garbage out), exercising, meditating, light therapy in the winter, minimizing some stress triggers, and some medication. So why, out of wisdom with a thread of fear, would I mess with any of it? I am not compulsive about any of this, but do believe steady keeps me mentally competitive. Notice I did not say "steady wins the race," for I have accepted my MI shadow, that my dear and fear-inducing Andy will be a passenger for life. It is not about winning or curing Andy, but accepting it as a lifelong battle for health and life itself. There is no finish line; Andy's shadow will follow me until I am "ashes to ashes, and dust to dust." To that reality, I now give Andy's shadow over my life the recognition it is due. Waging an open battle with my Mental Illness sounds much better than clinging to mental health in the shadows. I would rather be a warrior than a victim.

Most shy away from their own reality,
especially their feelings.
Life is such a wonderful journey as some say, but
that is hogwash, because in reality life is hard.
Feelings can be difficult and all consuming.
We see the pain as the enemy, but it is telling
us something. Wake up for there is something
wrong and it needs immediate attention.
Don't hide your pain, neither should
one wear it on one's sleeve.
In hiding from your pain, especially emotional
pain, the culture of "everything will work out" or
"it's all in God's plan" will destroy your reality.
You have a right to your pain, your reality.

The Reality
Mental Health Spectrum

Settle; calm down now. From the last chapter you might think that I believe Mental Illness is an ever-present burden and battle for life itself for everyone who suffers some of Andy's symptoms. Remember my diagnosis, label if you will, that I personally have accepted and owned – Major Depressive Disorder. Certainly not everyone who deals with Andy has a life-threateningly serious Mental Illness. On the other hand, others have a battle with Andy that is far more intense and debilitating than my own. Enter the concept of the Mental Health Spectrum; we all, as in ALL, fall on that spectrum. From total health to totally disabled mentally, and as I have alluded to before, it modulates for all of us as multiple factors in life change.

The breathing and respiratory example that follows has worked for me, so perhaps its breadth you will find usual as well. Some people suffer from a temporary viral cold, while others can get bronchitis or even pneumonia. Others suffer from allergies and asthma conditions. Sadly, people also cope with "major disorders" such as COPD and/or advanced stage lung cancer. If the analogy works, that is what I have experienced mentally – from an off day or short period of time to something major that has caused complete disorder in my life. Now there are factors in respiration, some under one's control and others of no fault of their own, that can bear on whether a viral cold can be more or less manageable for a period of time, to whether a person with an advanced respiratory condition like COPD or advanced lung cancer can cope for the rest of their lives. For example to name a few: did or does the person smoke; did or does the person work with toxic substances like asbestos; was the person born with a genetic/familial breathing disorder or disposition towards one; has the person or family taken mitigating steps to minimize exposure to allergens, bacteria, and viruses; what support system is in place while the person is ill; or how willing is or has the person been to incorporate diet, exercise, and medications into their treatment/coping plan. So true as well with Mental Illness, some things can be influenced readily, while others are out of anyone's control. Mix all these factors and more together that have a bearing on a person mentally, with the organ we call the brain that controls everything from physiology to the will to live, and you not only have complexity beyond imagination, but a spectrum from health to illness. A spectrum that spans living the dream and on cruise control to bracing for a crash and burn landing. All the while, one's Mental Health is fluctuating with the events and journey in life.

Anyone can read volumes of good research on Andy and the brain generally. I have read or browsed some topics, been in a couple treatment programs, and sat in enough counseling sessions to be aware and somewhat knowledgeable. With that said, there are three truths I know for myself currently. First, all the research and studies on Andy and Mental Health form a useful background. Second, no one can tell me for sure what the answer is for my Mental Health because of the complexity of the brain and life generally. Finally, in dealing with my Mental Illness, the essence of who I am as a human being and my relation to others has come into sharper focus. To this last statement I now turn for the remainder of the book. As stated before, there is no magic pill, or secret sauce that keeps me flying and not in the direction of the cuckoo's nest. But what I can offer is what has fueled my current flight and my will to keep my life's journey aloft.

Truly looking in the mirror and accepting
one's reflection is a brave act.
Show up and love yourself. Show up, and
listen to other's sacred story as well. Especially
when it is embarrassing and/or painful.
Trying is not the goal, maybe a start at best.
The doing is what leads to being.

Body

Show up - Faith

Faith is a belief. When your mind tells you the exact opposite with a Mental Illness, you have to believe that it is an issue of the brain organ, that it is multi-faceted, AND that the body has a tremendous ability to heal if given half a chance. The mind will tell you otherwise: in depression, to not show up at all and hide; in anxiety to panic/run/avoid; and unavoidably at times and for some, the mind tells you the way out is to not show up at all anymore, literally, as in suicide. In my worst mental condition, I never had a plan, but did have suicidal ideations. And yes, death or any effect it would have on my loved ones did not matter. And in that type of despair, it was the most maddening for me when you realize the love that you have for a spouse, friend, child, or grandchild cannot make you rally. The end is all-too near.

As I have been there, in such a state, more than once, my call is for the mentally distressed to show up with every fiber of their being. That means get up and drag oneself out of bed. Get out and drag oneself out for a short walk. Answer calls and messages, and be brutally honest with your current state with those who love you. There will be time to process the confusion, guilt, and even shame later; now your life is at stake. This brings me to the second way to show up and have faith. At this degree of distress, one must swallow any sense of pride and put oneself in the hands of a loved one or medical facility/counselor/ emergency department. Show up, state that you are desperate, and put yourself in the care of another.

For friends and loved ones, the message is the same – show up. No matter what the person in a mental crisis says, does, or does not do. No matter whether you think you have nothing to say or offer. The one in mental distress may do anything from avoiding you, belittle your effort, to outright yell and scream at you. Show up anyway. They are not in their right mind and are judging themselves and may likely do so with you as well. Still show up. When someone is thrashing around in the water with a chance of drowning, a person needs to show up or it may be all over. Prepare yourself for the "thrashing" around; remember showing up is not only an act of courage in this situation, but an act of compassion. You do not need to say much, just as a person thrashing around in the water does not need advice and counseling at the moment. By your simple presence, volumes will be spoken and the person in distress will be distracted for a period, and will know that you empathize with them no matter what they say at the time. Frankly, for that period of time, self-harm to the point of suicide can be delayed and potentially averted.

Finally, while there are no easy answers, society-at-large and the medical profession needs to show up more in a big way. Show up with resources and personnel. Amidst the good work that far too few are doing in this regard, the body of work and effort on behalf of Mental Illness is lacking. Showing up with judgment, shaming, and/or ridicule of the mentally distressed does not help. Blaming the mentally ill for anything from gun violence to too much stress on our social support systems is not productive. Instead of thinking of financial gain and/ or strain, the medical and pharmaceutical community should show up with the empathy, compassion, and resources to match not only the current situation, but match their oaths and creeds to which they vow or aspire. I repeat, in a way, what I stated earlier in the book: when it comes to the beating heart, the breathing lungs, bowels and bladders, balls and breasts, a thunderous response comes forth. For the mentally ill and distressed, a whisper is heard in comparison from the medical profession, and from society-at-large from which it flows. Yes, if only. If only we put as much effort and empathy toward the brain as we do other body parts.

We often take for granted that when the mind speaks,
the body will follow. There is wisdom in understanding
that when the body speaks, the mind will follow as well.
Listening is not leaving a lasting
impression or fixing someone.
As difficult as it seems, silence speaks volumes and can give hope.

Mind

Listen - Hope

It was very interesting when I looked up others' wisdom from quotes on listening and the mind, as I found almost nothing. There was plenty to scan on listening to your body, but not the mind. There was also plenty available on speaking your mind or letting your heart speak, but not listening. While I did not do an exhaustive search, I found this insightful. We find it natural and wise to pay attention to what our body is telling us, but not to the mind that runs everything. If I have a twinge in my back here or there, I should listen to what my body is telling me. A numbness in my left arm, and I should pay attention and get it checked out in case it is anything from a pinched nerve to a heart attack. But have a flat period emotionally, sullen stretch, or a sadness that just does not seem to break, and the advice is not about awareness or listening typically, but to do something – snap out of it or pull yourself up by your bootstraps. The other tendency is dismissiveness or to depend on the "if only": nothing can be that bad, if only I had a vacation, better spouse, another job, etc. I do not mean to belittle the attempts at doing something, changing something, or cheering oneself up, but they all have little to do with truly listening to the state of one's mind.

There is such a thing, listening to one's mind, that originates in Eastern traditions primarily, and some Western contemplative traditions as well. Words and phrases such as mindfulness, meditation, prayer, and emptying one's thoughts come to mind. Having been exposed to breathing techniques of Hatha Yoga over 20 years ago, and more intentionally during my Mental Health relapses while in the programs I was in, I have come to incorporate and find beneficial the use of such techniques, whether of the mind only or with physicality, such as yoga/stretching positions.

Here, I am not giddy with advice, as in, "You gotta try this or that," but for me it seems logical. For the body, sleep/rest is necessary for recovery/rejuvenation. So true for the mind as well. For the body, it is also suggested to not only exercise but to stretch as well. Why? For flexibility, pliability, and injury prevention. So true for the mind as well? Beyond sleep, it would seem useful in order to prevent injury to allow for and practice pliability, awareness, and flexibility of the mind.

The most basic concept of mindfulness for me is, "I am not my thoughts," but they can drive and dictate my life completely and potentially destructively if not attended to. As a technique example, I sit quietly in a semi-reclined chair (for my back comfort) with headphones on with soft instrumental music. Next, I envision that I am sitting by a quiet stream or lake. Why? Because it comes easily to mind, as in very real, given the lakes and streams I have taken breaks beside on my bicycle and fishing trips. I can "see" it in my mind with little effort. Just described is the "physicality" of the technique. The mind part starts with concentrating on my belly breathing as if following it on a wave. Then I just allow thoughts, any thoughts, to come. When they do, I visualize them on a leaf upstream coming towards me. I focus on the thought intently as it comes close and then just watch it pass and drift away.

At times, the same thought comes back over and over again, and that's okay. Sometimes a thought comes to mind and I never get to focus on it, much less let it drift away, because another thought takes center stream. That's fine too. When it feels too chaotic and confusing, I return to floating on the wave of my belly breathing. The length of time can vary, from "why bother" short to half an hour.

The point? To quiet the mind, and awareness through deliberate practice and effort. In doing so, I have learned that thoughts are just thoughts, and they become more sticky and potentially dangerous by what we do consciously or unconsciously, by giving them added weight and meaning. By practicing the conscious side of the mindfulness equation, I have found that I have become more aware when I have unconsciously given added emphasis to certain thoughts. I am careful here to not say "control" over my thoughts, but awareness. Thoughts come and go, at times with little or no warning; control is limited but awareness is possible.

So, what does all this have to do with the last topic of this chapter's trilogy – Hope? Everything. To use it as an acronym:

- **H**esitation: Attending to your mind regularly gives a person the skills to stop and hesitate in the moment, and as often as necessary, amidst significant mental distress; when the brain goes into a spin cycle, flush cycle, or a near death spiral.
- **O**penness: As a body can open its arms for more, the mind is open to more than spin, flush and death when they scream for attention and dominance.
- **P**ossible: You train yourself that there is more; you believe it to the core of your being when the cycles and spiral become entrenched and chronic.
- **E**ffort: Practicing using your mind in a pliable and flexible way, with focus and calm, will prove invaluable when every ounce of effort, if not life-saving effort, will be demanded amidst significant mental distress.

"'You shall not take vengeance, nor bear any grudge
against the children of your people; but you shall
love your neighbor as yourself." - Leviticus 19:18
"You shall love your neighbor as yourself."
Mark 12:31, Matthew 22:39, Luke 10:27

Spirit
Divine Spark – Love

The concept of Spirit circulates in conversations, ranging from pure hogwash to the divine and everything in between. Ethereal, no question. Philosophical, for sure. Can't be proven, you can bet your periodic table on it. Not being a philosopher, nor a social anthropologist, does not prevent me from understanding that from the dawn of human consciousness, we humans have been on a quest for the purpose in life and death, while along the way succeeding and failing at loving ourselves and not killing each other. The above quotes come from the two of the three monotheistic traditions I am most familiar with: Judaism and Christianity.

First, I know for sure there is me, and also you/others. Second, in the midst of Mental Illness for me, God as believed and portrayed as a divine essence, is NOT the issue. This reminds me of an iconic TV ad or movie depiction of a relationship, when a passerby first hears a thud followed by a loud crash. The person looks up and sees a woman throwing belongings (likely a boyfriend's) out of a second story window while cursing the former loved one's and God's name in the same sentence with each toss. Just envision the same as true for me with God during a Mental Health relapse; out the window goes God, grace, faith, hope, and love. But there is no thud or loud crash, any passerby might just shake their head and think, "What's up with Mick?" When I have lost my true self, and in grasping for it with as much certainty as a firm grasp on air, I lose much of my outward thinking towards others, and have little or no time for the philosophical otherness of God. I am no longer my true self during a relapse when Andy takes full control of the wheel; I no longer love myself, hope has turned to shame, and faith being fleeting would be an exaggeration.

So where, might you ask, is the positive and the promise in this chapter as this section approaches its final approach? Are you ready...well here it is...it's a mystery. Why am I still here, when during my relapses I have suicidal ideations? Why am I still here, when thousands of others annually commit suicide due to Mental Illness and distress? Why has my wife, Rita, stayed with me and my children still loved me, when for considerable lengths of time during a relapse, I don't even want to hang out with myself? Why do I go into a relapse of, and as mysteriously come out of, a relapse in mental health? If God is a mystery, so, too, is the brain, at least at this point in history. Sure, there are hints for me, such as family genetics, the lack of light in the winter, brain chemistry alterations, etc., but they are semi-solid ingredients at best, certainly not as solid as concrete.

While a mystery, my answer is that I have been fortunate, lucky even, and for this I am indeed grateful. I am no stronger or weaker, faith filled or not, courageous or cowardly, than all those presently suffering from Mental Illness or the countless numbers who have killed themselves due to severe mental distress. Along with mystery and good fortune, I fall on the concept of love. Love not as a warm fuzzy or erotic feeling, but one of sacrificial and unconditional giving of oneself to another. When I have felt, during a relapse, all the emotions about myself, except love, I have clung to the belief that I am worthy of respect – that this episode, this relapse, is largely not of my own doing. When others could just as easily, if not reasonably, cut and run, they still have loved me when I am "out of my mind." For this I am grateful the most. Finally, I believe that in the human condition, there is the mystery of love itself, God if you will, that sacrifices and binds us together against all odds and adversities, when we are open to being the best version of ourselves.

To this I have now come, to the concept of Spirit, soul, or divine spark, as I call it. In the tradition that I know best, Christianity, it is said that God is love. If God is love, then Jesus was/is the fullest embodiment and model of what unconditional and sacrificial love is, and the Spirit is the potential that each of us can be guided by that type of love each day of our life. To this end, love of self, love of others, and love as a mystery beyond our understanding, is our life's purpose and journey.

I am okay with this truth being a mystery for me;
a divine spark, the soul, and being Spirit driven by love.

SECTION FOUR

LifeSavers

"You're Going to Jump Out of a Perfectly Good Airplane?!"

Over ten years ago, a colleague and co-worker at Hastings Family Service was approaching a milestone birthday and decided she wanted to tandem parachute with an instructor out of an airplane. The only catch? She wanted someone else to go with her. I volunteered readily; it was on my bucket list. If asked the question at the top or similar, I would simply answer, "Yep, why not?" By voice, or the look on the face of those I told, the major sentiment was, "Are you out of your mind?" While it did not make me reconsider, it did make me think about the small risk I was taking with my life, and that I would most likely be scared out of my jumpsuit just before the jump.

The weekend came, and some supporters of us (family and friends) came to the jump site near Hammond WI to watch us take off and land. After the usual jump instructions and suiting up, we both said our "see you in a while" with a wink, and loaded the airplane which took off with 10,000 feet as the objective. A final group encouragement and pep talk by the jump leader took place at that altitude, and then we clipped up to our jump instructor. Approaching the open door of the airplane with my instructor attached behind me, a sickening feeling came over me just before we mostly rolled forward out of the plane. The first second or two was absolutely sickening and terror filled, but then with no close frame of reference to trigger my sense of falling, the feeling went immediately away; free fall was indeed freeing. Then the parachute was opened with a sensation of an abrupt stop, which felt like being launched upwards; stomach in throat-sort of stuff, but then the slow float began which calmed my insides. That is until the instructor decided, unbeknownst to me, to pull on his control ropes and do 360 spins first one way then another. Until we landed, I felt I was going to "toss my cookies," which was followed by disorientation while walking back to the hanger. My co-worker on the other hand had the opposite experience with her instructor; slow float down with no spinning, and the instructor even let her pull on the control ropes to do slow turns.

I use this as an analogy of sorts with my experience of and personal awareness of Mental Illness. Andy has come beckoning for me to make that jump into the terror of severe mental distress a number of times. Yes, out of one's mind, is an apt description for what then takes place. As I roll into depression and/or anxiety, it is indeed sickening and terror filled; "oh no, here we go again." But unlike the free fall of parachuting, mainly doom and gloom clouds my perspective while free falling into relapse. Nothing, and I mean nothing including how many times I have gone through it before, has prepared me for the abrupt and halting thoughts to just stop and end it all. If not suicidal ideation, few things seem to be normal; uncontrolled spinning is a good analogy. Eventually, mysteriously, luckily, and with good medical intervention, I have hit solid ground again. But when first into recovery, there is a considerable period of time when I feel a bit weak and unsettled by it all.

Three items I leave with you as landing this flight into the cuckoo's nest is upon us: Trust, Presence, and Humor.

I have no knowledge of airplanes or parachutes, but I trust that they will work. Even though shaken in a relapse, I trust the vast majority of mechanics and mechanisms that are along for my flight; the psychiatrists, nurses, and therapists of all kinds and the mechanisms of in-patient wards as well as out-patient programming. When you can't fly your own plane of life, it is best to put it in the hands of professionals. Sure, I have been critical of pieces of the mental health care industry in this book; as with almost any plane, flight plan, or flight itself, it could be better and smoother.

Yes, there have been 360 spins with friends and relatives on my flights. They have been anywhere from totally absent, to insensitive or ignorant, during my fall into depression and anxiety. My experiences have taught me to cling to, and show honest gratitude for, those who loved me when I took flight and who also greeted me the same on landing. They were bewildered and near helpless to assist me as they watched me take flight into the cuckoo's nest; but they are the ones who have loved me through thick and thick, they are made of the right stuff. As stated in the beginning, I felt lonely but was not alone. When wanting to hide in depression or run away during high anxiety, I know from wisdom now, to not only welcome, but ask for their loving presence.

Finally, one of my best litmus tests for my current mental health, and certainly when walking away from a flight into the cuckoo's nest, is humor. When I found that I could laugh, smile, and appreciate a good joke, I knew I was in a good or better place mentally. My most memorable dialogue, the only one I remember from the parachute jump, was from the jump leader just moments before we all jumped out of that perfectly good airplane. After the last-minute instructions, he offered anyone who wanted one, a LifeSaver mint. Playing to the moment and irony does not do it justice. As freaked out as I was becoming, I appreciated the gesture and took my LifeSaver to chew on. So true was it with my wife and family, friends, and professionals all along my journey with Andy and flights into the cuckoo's nest; simple humor, and appreciation of it, has been a sign of hope and health.

Wheels down, good and faith filled virtual passengers on this flight. My only advice, whether you are facing Andy yourself, much less the cuckoo's nest, or assisting someone in that type of flight in life is:

Accept the lifesavers
Whether solo or in great sum
Medical, loved ones, or humor
Matters not whence they come

Trust
- Self
- Loved Ones
- Professionals

MICK HUMBERT

Presence
- To Self
- To Others
- To Fellow Warriors

Humor
- Walk lightly
- Enter lightly
- Exit lightly

BICYCLES BUILT
FOR THE BLUES

Foreword...143
Absolute...147

Frame...149
Andy and Andrea's Frame 155
Decals that Stick... 157
A Bit Sticky.. 165
Deflating...167
Weight, No Wait!..171
Living on the Edge..174
Cadence 178
The Finish Line? 186
Mirrors.. 190
Pedals.. 193
Shoo-es 196
Seat 199
Handlebars... 202
Derailleur.. 205
Cell Phone 208
Flats 211
Riding in a Pack 214
Drafting 217
Solo Riding 221
Time to Ride.. 224

Dedication

To the family and friends
who visited me during my
three inpatient Mental Health stays
during the winter of 2017,
and the patients, yes warriors,
that were there at the same time
as I was.

To all the staff who engage in dignifying and serving
residents well at the Senior Assisted Living
and Long-Term Care facility where I am a Chaplain.

FOREWORD

It's baaaaaack!!! To wake up at 3:00 AM one December 8th morning (2016) with a heightened level of anxiety, of which I had instant recognition from 25-30 years ago, was disturbing to say the least. The downward spiral ensued quickly and I was in a mental health unit within 3 weeks. I spent Christmas with strangers, each of whom had their own mental health crisis, where lack of privacy was the rule with constant background noise, little view of the outside world, and being locked-up with your shoelaces and belt taken away from you as a norm. Six months later, I am writing this book, having written 22 poems as a cathartic memory of my journey and only six weeks out of being in my last inpatient stay. At its worst, I wanted my life over with, although I never formulated a suicidal plan. When your wife, kids, and grandchildren cannot hold up your willingness to live anymore, you are in a very dark, humiliating, and guilt-ridden place.

This is not the typical beginning of a book. As the word "foreword" implies, I am going to be upfront, brutally honest, and forward from the get-go. I have suffered from a Mental Illness, disease if you will, since I was at least 30 years old when my physical health deteriorated due to a back disability. Cause and effect would be a stretch, but saying that chronic pain exacerbated my genetic/familial predisposition toward a condition some thirty years later, classified as Bipolar II, would be true in my opinion. Once titled Agitative Depression, a generalized anxiety disorder (GAD) presents itself, along with seasonal affective disorder (SAD) in my case, coupled with a chronic back condition to an extent that the result can be deep depression driven by anxiety.

Some 25-30 years ago, I was under the delusion that with some moderate dosage of anti-anxiety and antidepressant medications, I could "handle it" or that I was "scot-free." Wrong. Chronic pain, GAD, and SAD as a trifecta is a wicked and brutally disabling, and even life-threatening combination which I will live with and hopefully manage the rest of my life. That honest assessment and acceptance has come over a recent five-month battle with this major depressive disorder, which included my previous medication of 25 years "crapping out," as they call it, three visits of about a week each to hospital inpatient mental health units, and two-day treatment programs to deal with a crisis resulting from high anxiety, depression, and suicidal ideation.

It's never coming back!!! I am a Chaplain at an Assisted Living and Long-Term Care Facility. I find parallels with the lives of residents to the crisis I went through; both triumphs and challenges. I will never say that I understand their situation completely, and certainly will not claim to understand how they feel. But the potential for aloneness and loneliness, as well as anxiety and depression are a reality for some of the residents. The sense of loss, and of no hope for turning back is palpable. I manage an illness that can cause self-isolation, anxiety, and depression, while ministering to a segment of residents where those are present as well. Comparing Mental Illness and aging in an assisted living residence must be done with nuance and care. I have chosen to stay away from direct comparisons through the use of an item everyone can relate to, a bicycle.

In the ensuing chapters, I will build a bicycle, using the relatively common understanding of bicycle components and their purpose as analogies for the difficult topics of depression and anxiety, as well as aging and decline, that I will explore. As with my previous books, I will begin each chapter with a verse or two from the World English Bible translation of Christian Scripture. The bicycle component analogy will explore not only the horror of the Mental Illness, but the help that is available as well. Having gone through two outpatient programs, I borrow some of that insight, namely from dialectic behavioral therapy (DBT) and cognitive behavioral therapy (CBT). Of course, I am writing now entering firmly into restorative health, so the raw and visceral emotions related to the disease will be diluted somewhat. However, all the poems were written during my last inpatient mental health stay or during the last day treatment immediately afterward, over a five-week period. The edginess and stark reality of the disease I suffer from is best seen then in the poetry; the remainder of the writing are reflections from hindsight. For residents in Assisted Living and Long-Term Care, my thoughts and insights come from residents themselves, staff, and my own observations. I have found that I must honor Mental Illness and decline with aging as much on their own terms as possible. These reflections are cathartic and a launch point to moving forward in life. It is important to distinguish between Mick who manages Bipolar II (hindsight in relative health in the narrative) from Mick as Bipolar II (in the throes of the disease in the poetry). It is equally important not to stereotype senior residents. While the challenges to mind, body, and spirit are certainly evident and widespread, many residents travel this journey of life with great grace and purpose.

Having biked a recumbent seriously for some 30 years now as one means of coping with my back disability and Mental Illness, I know pretty well the mechanics of putting together this bike. However, you learn and are assisted by others in your travels through life. In particular, I wish to acknowledge the important role this time around that my family and friends were in standing in a Mental Health crisis with me - you know who you are. Finally, as vague, confusing, and ill-refined as the mental health service field is at times, numerous therapists, counselors, social workers, nurses, psychiatrists, and yes patients, were along for my recent bumpy Mental Illness ride. To and for them, the memory is strong. Likewise, the many residents and staff where I work are a wealth of wisdom, courage, and integrity from whom I have benefited greatly.

So, I am ready to proceed, and if you are, read along as I build bicycles built for the blues. Bring a wrench because some of what follows is gut-wrenching. A hammer will come in handy as the disease and aging hammer a person into submission too. Ooh, and bring some grease and oil for the later chapters because in both cases life can run smoothly. As cathartically reflective as this writing has been for me, any insight or benefit you gain from reading it, I consider an honor.

ABSOLUTE

From last Mental Illness
As inpatient – acute
Six weeks later
More balanced – more astute

During that time
22 poems did compute
My truth, my illness
Of my mind no longer mute

Normalcy returning,
Chaplaincy as work too
Pondering elderly resident parallels
In more than just a few

While the bicycle
Holds together this route
poetry shows most clearly
MI as a brute

Wonder – increasing health
My writing may dilute
How depression and anxiety
Can be absolute

Not a scholarly exam
Which specialist could dispute
Just visceral and raw
My journey – others, nothing cute

Success to me
If only a bit to commute
Bad MI and elderly stereotypes
From huge to minute

So I build a bicycle
To inform not distribute
better understanding
I wish to contribute

End of the second week of May 2017
Final Poem

Matthew 7:24-27

"Everyone therefore who hears these words of mine and does them, I will liken him to a wise man who built his house on a rock. ^{25} The rain came down, the floods came, and the winds blew and beat on that house; and it didn't fall, for it was founded on the rock. ^{26} Everyone who hears these words of mine and doesn't do them will be like a foolish man who built his house on the sand. ^{27} The rain came down, the floods came, and the winds blew and beat on that house; and it fell—and its fall was great."

Frame

"You get what you get, and don't throw a fit"

The beginning of any bicycle necessitates discussion of the frame; what type of tubing and the angles will go a long way in determining the strength, stiffness, longevity, and comfort of the bike. Way back in the 90s and before, it was all about steel alloys. Aluminum framing took hold after that, with even some composite materials. The expensive rage now is ultralight carbon fiber frames. While frames come in all makes, models, and sizes, understanding at least what you have or do not have can prove helpful in determining how one must ride and what one might expect from the bicycle.

The analogy to oneself is that by genetics and environment your frame has largely been built and it will be the frame you live with the rest of your life. Accepting one's framework, while difficult at times, can prove helpful in traversing life with some wisdom and grace. We each have the parents and upbringing we had, and its effects on us are both positive and negative. Our body chemistry, the brain in particular for Mental Illness, is largely genetic and inherited; how your "brain is wired" as the saying goes. Finally, our life's experiences puts our framework or frame of reference to the test over time. Sure, we can adapt and change somewhat, but the predominant reality is that we will function our entire lives with the frame that has been inherited or experientially fixed. Radical swap outs for an entirely different frame of reference or framework from which we function or see the world, while not entirely impossible, is rare in my opinion.

What I believe I have, how I am built, is a combination of Bipolar II (agitative depression), SAD (seasonal affective disorder), and multiple thoracic disc damage and resultant chronic pain. The acronym I call my "friend" is ANDY: AN for anxiety, D for depression, and Y for daily. For better or worse, it is how I am built; chronic back pain poking and prodding at anxiety and depression is not a healthy frame of reference from which to live, much less thrive. At least that has been my personal experience.

So if we get what we get, the question is how much of a "fit are we going to throw" physically, mentally, and emotionally in objection to the built-in essence of who we are. In the world of Mental Illness, I have experienced in myself three choices: ignore (your frame) the way you are, wish you were something else (had a different frame), or accept the way you are and move forward. Ignoring the potential danger in the way I am built is how I would characterize my approach when things are going good, fine, OK, or at least sub-acute. You ignore the warning signs, take things for granted, and are not on the look-out for the big potholes in your life's journey. I would eat and sleep as I would like, exercise less than more, let my introversion isolate myself, and count on the anxiety and depression medication cocktail way too much to keep things under control.

What happened 25-30 years ago and then in the last year was exactly this lack of diligence to how I am built to operate, combined with an increase in outward stresses (new job, more hours, more responsibility) and inward stresses (the medication "pooped out" and became ineffective). SNAP. NOT AGAIN!! My mental health and ability to cope was quickly flushed down the toilet, I fell off the MI cliff, or as they referred to me when I checked myself into an inpatient mental health ward for the first time in December 2016, I have a "major depressive disorder." Try swallowing that trifecta and digest it for a while and see what that does for your sense of ego, and self-worth: first its "major," and second a want to avoid and hide, if not wanting to be dead level of "depression," and finally there is nothing orderly about it anymore, you are "disordered." The second choice in dealing with my framework, my mind, my inner self was to go acute when things fell apart; I wanted out of it and now!! I wanted a different frame, and cried out that the storm I was riding through was unfair. What did I do to deserve this? Why can't I have my old self back? Please, give me the drug, the combo, the magic elixir to make it all go away! I tried to exercise, eat, and sleep my way out of it as a panic-induced solution. Striving and thriving go out the window, while purely animalistic survival enters with a mind not able to assist much, and a will that turns to suicidal ideation as a seemingly reasonable option. Will someone, anyone, give me a different frame to ride; because I wouldn't wish this ride on my worst enemy!!

There is a saying, "The mind is a terrible thing to waste." But what do you do when the mind itself is in a wasteland of anxious and depressed emotions; when you can't think your way out of a paper bag. Unlike the black-and-white view of a life built on rock or sand in the above-mentioned verses from the gospel of Matthew, what if you have no real choice and the slippery sandy slope of Mental Illness is all you have to work with? The mostly ignorant misunderstandings of American society toward Mental Illness do not help much either. Have you beat it yet? Are you over it yet? Are you crazy? Oh, so you needed to go to the nuthouse? Why don't you just pull yourself up by the britches? Your faith in God is being tested, you will be a better person for it afterward.

What follows is my experience only, and certainly not meant to be a how-to-book your way out of Mental Illness. There is so much we don't know about the brain and Mental Illness; how the mind can be diseased with no apparent pathology to point to (yet). There is enough known about the framework of the mind by therapy and pharmacology to take educated guesses, like throwing darts at a dartboard, that by the way, is at a considerable distance away. I can point to contributing factors but I am still bewildered and amazed at how the severe MI episode starts and how seemingly I have come out of it each time. My opinion is when the mental health experts are honest, they don't know exactly why either.

So I can't ignore the frame I have; I can't replace it either. As a saying goes, "bloom where you are planted." But how do I do that when I don't want anything to do with this particular garden? So let us begin, as I lay before you my experiences in the midst of a MI crisis during the winter of 2017. As stated in the foreword, pay close attention to the poetry as they were all written either during the MI crisis or during the initial few weeks of recovery. There will be sadness and hope, desperation and inspiration in the following pages. So, saddle up, if you will, bring plenty of water and some rain gear, because this ride is exhausting and stormy much of the time.

This is a Recording (Gehenna)

A depository near Jerusalem
Where garbage and animals did burn
And unclean corpses too
Out of derision and to spurn

Does such a living hell
Analogy to compare
Humans suffering today
Now death do stare?

Avoiding and ruminating
Back for round two
Anxiety and depression
One hellish bitter stew

Supposedly not my fault
Imbalance of the brain
When hope and joy cease
Entereth self-disdain

First the shock
Hideous return
Not again!
Another turn?!

Grin for awhile
A front, a denial
When bear it no more
Death's thoughts do file

Makes no sense
A life seemingly so true
Love, support and good habits
Still breached by the blues

Loss of self
core slipping away
The multi-headed symptoms
Now here to stay?

Your mind and body
Assailed and terrorized
Losing battle played out
Behind my very eyes

Tried so hard
Then guilt set in
Presence to loving family
Future fading thin

To start another chapter
First turn the page
Inpatient Mental Health
Inner self to gauge

Hanging by a thread
Or the tip of my last spoon
Will this turned page
Offer some hope soon?

3rd Inpatient Treatment in four months
End of March 2017

Andy and Andrea's Frame

In Senior Living Residency, the frame of reference, I suggest, is a box; an ever increasingly small box as incapacitation of body, mind, and/or spirit takes place. Confinement of all three is one of the real but often unspoken realities. "You have to assume as a baseline that everyone who lives here doesn't want to be here." That is a close approximation of what one lead manager of the senior living facility I work at stated. The following are some ways I suggest residents get boxed in when they call a senior living residence their home:

- Personal choice changes
- Personal relationships are interrupted or lost
- Comfort food – surroundings – bed – noises all change
- You literally live in a box; a coffin-like reality where they will eventually wheel you out in a bag from one box or another.
- You become the served, not needed anymore; with increasing incapacitation, most things are either provided for you or directly done for or to you.
- Loneliness or aloneness increases even when surrounded by people.
- It can become difficult to find purpose, hope, and meaning for life.
- The potential reality of anxiety and/or depression prowls the hallways and howls within many souls.

Andy moved from assisted living to TCU briefly and then into long term care. Andy was full of life and purpose when he had his "A game" in the outside world. He would be the great friend, a spark in any gathering, quite the ladies man, and the loved patriarch of a family. For a period of time while more independent in assisted living, Andy transferred his zest for life to others around him; he sang and told jokes, while engaging with anyone and everyone. Brightness and joy oozed from him as he took great pride in taking care of others often by simply cheering them up. When I saw him in TCU, things had changed; illness and dysfunction had come visiting. At times, I would hear him say the end was coming with a sadness that defied his usual persona. Then, a partial rebound from the ailments brought back some of his intrigue and purpose for living. Andy increasingly knows that, in his 90's, the end is near. As a faith filled man, I do not sense that a fear of dying is as much of an issue as is losing his joyful ability to live, for he loves it so much.

Andrea lives in one of the memory units, where the individuals managing the milder stages of Dementia and Alzheimer's live. The family was very attentive and caring about the transition for Andrea; as a chaplain they stated her faith life was important and hoped we could provide some comfort for her. I first had interactions with Andrea when she was wandering up and down the halls. I reintroduced myself to her, and asked her if I could assist in some way. She had her purse in hand and said she was going to the parking lot to get into her car to go home. She had visited this hotel long enough and it was time to go. With some prompting, I brought her back to her room where her familiar items and some furniture were. She calmed down some and said this was her bedroom and was willing to stay for a while. In future visits, Andrea was cognitive enough to talk about her husband who had passed and how she wished she would die and go be with him as there was not much left for her now. This would become her mantra. Even as she faithfully would be brought to worship service, she engaged in little else that was offered; occasional family and staff visits surrounded by an aloneness and loneliness for her husband.

Psalm 22:1-2
My God, my God, why have you forsaken me?
Why are you so far from helping me, and
from the words of my groaning?
My God, I cry in the daytime, but you don't answer;
in the night season, and am not silent.

Decals that Stick

The make and model of my bicycle frame has been established as being Bipolar II with Seasonal Affective Disorder and chronic pain from multiple thoracic disc ruptures. With any bike, the decals add to the story: Schwinn, Giro, Specialized, Shimano, Cervelo, Trek, etc. So also true with Mental Illness and the stickers that remain in my memory; some old and some new, but certainly a permanent mark on life's memory and journey. So, what Mental Health decals stick out in my memory at this writing?

A sampling of my Mental Health Decals – Old to New that stick
(a chronology of sorts)

It sticks – 30 years ago when I woke up one December day to get ready for work and could not turn easily side to side. The frustration and effort to overcome daily chronic pain that ensued is one of my most visible decals marking my life's journey. It brought me out of my first profession as a Dentist, it exhausted me emotionally and spiritually, it brought me literally to my knees.

It sticks - maintaining the quality of my dental work (let's say B+ average) while I trashed my emotional wellbeing (enter high anxiety and depression).

It sticks - many nights 20-30 years ago that I would be overcome with emotion and get up out of bed to cry in another room so as not to disturb my wife, Rita.

It sticks - changing everything possible in my Dental profession for 10 years to maintain my practice. I eventually settled on only 3-4 hours 3 mornings a week, sort of pretending to still have a practice because I did not see any other option at the time.

It sticks - falling to my knees in front of my wife, balling my eyes out and her suggesting for the first time that I see a therapist. I remember how my socially conditioned self felt when I drove myself to a therapist for the first time and waited in the waiting room.

It sticks - feeling absolutely guilt-ridden for not being able to hold up my end of the deal as husband and father of two young children.

It sticks – going for lonely walks of only one mile and feeling frustrated and dejected that my back ached so much.

It sticks – the time I called into a crisis line and discussion I had over having suicidal thoughts but no plan.

It sticks – after one such walk, and the emotional grip I lost, when I experienced my first panic attack and began hyperventilating.

It sticks – taking the MMPI for the first time and being told I was clinically depressed.

It sticks – understanding a solution/answer is typically more than one thing, and going to all kinds of specialists looking for an answer: Orthopedic surgeon, Neurosurgeon, Chiropractor, Acupuncturist, Allergist, Osteopaths and Physical Trainer.

It sticks – after an orthopedic surgeon giving me the option of back surgery for the neurosurgeon and my own investigation discovering how invasive the surgery would be with only a 50-50 chance of making any improvement in pain.

It sticks – the neurosurgeon stating quite bluntly that I shouldn't want this type of thoracic back surgery unless I couldn't walk or was peeing on the floor from effects of direct spinal cord impingement.

It sticks – being so emotionally stressed while trying to do dentistry, that when I gave a lower mandibular block injection to a patient who flinched, that I flinched as well.

It sticks – the conclusion I came to after suffering in dental practice for 10 years to give up on my profession that I worked so hard to achieve.

It sticks – my first go-round with antidepressants was Prozac and losing 8 pounds in three days due to night sweats. I was giving a little presentation at a staff meeting and could think what I wanted to say, but could not speak effectively as I wanted. The ethics of practicing dentistry in such a state dictated to me that I should and did discontinue taking Prozac.

It sticks – the conversation I had with my brother and father who I was in dental practice with, when I cried telling them I was giving up Dentistry.

It sticks – the benefit of my first therapist, Mark, who listened through my processing my family upbringing and decision to give up dental practice. On telling me that through this whole process I had been making good decisions and saying, "Mick, if you told me that your next decision was to go to Nepal and see a guru, and he told you to eat lama shit, I would trust you at this point." I remembered I laughed and knew that some hope for normalcy had returned.

It sticks – when sitting against a wall in my young daughter Teresa's bedroom to cry after my wife went off to work, when this young two-year-old came into the room without my knowing it, put her hand on my shoulder and said, "It will be OK daddy."

It sticks – after giving up patient practice, doing some book and HR type work in the basement at the Dental office since I didn't know what else to do.

It sticks – after having given up dentistry, and making the decision to go big time into careful physical training to strengthen my back and discovering while in training that if I rode a recumbent stationary bike it did not exacerbate my back pain.

It sticks – one winter when even after giving up dentistry that I had such an anxiety attack that I told my wife I did not feel safe and called for an emergency county crisis intervention. Two ladies came over, and I remember telling them that "going to the dental office was like going to an accident scene with yellow tape around it." Her answer really stuck, "If it is that bad, then why do you keep going back." I decided to leave the family practice completely shortly thereafter.

It sticks – the fall that I got my first recumbent bike, a red long wheelbase Ryan with under the seat steering. I was serious about testing out the next spring whether recumbent bicycling would be my one main physical outlet I could do with no back pain.

It sticks – after going to a specialist who did a myelogram of four thoracic discs telling me that all four were ruptured and no need to test even further. He told me I was lucky that I did not have surgery when the only MRI result going into a decision was one herniated disc > that intervention would likely have been a never-ending cascade of increasing back problems.

It sticks – that finding out what was wrong with my back after 10+ years of suffering in pain felt like a relief. Knowing what you are up against is some comfort.

It sticks – another tough winter when I biked a few times, at least once each month, when the weather was in the mid-30's and the shoulders were clear and having about 2 hours of mental clarity and feeling normal in my own skin. I knew at that point that there was a biochemical possibility of some mental normalcy I could achieve due to this endorphin-type experiment.

It sticks – on my third therapist/psychiatrist when I told her of this seeming winter pattern and presently going through a tough winter emotionally again, that she apologized for a diagnosis of SAD never being considered before while in therapy. The therapy and pharmacological decision was to increase antidepressant drug therapy (Paxil and Wellbutrin) along with light therapy in the winter.

It sticks – the near normal feeling I had on Paxil for over 15 years. In that relative state of mental health I changed careers twice, became a deacon in the Catholic Church followed by a Master's degree. I increasingly became an avid recumbent cyclist to the extent that I have ridden in every state, and done 10 fundraising rides over 10 years while raising $100,000 for various charities.

It sticks – in hindsight that the riding, including two cross-country rides and Alaska/Yukon, while for enjoyment and altruism, were also to prove something to myself – that I was good enough even amidst the backpedaling I did in Mental Health and professional careers.

It sticks – the tiredness and sexual dysfunction produced by Paxil that I did not like but tolerated.

It sticks – this past fall (2016) deciding without doctor's advice, after being on my typical low dose of summer Paxil, to try getting off Paxil and just stay/increase Wellbutrin to compensate for my usual winter dose.

It sticks – December 8th, 2016 while on vacation in Florida having a great time, waking up at 3:00 am for a brief bit with that all too familiar anxiety feeling from the past. It got progressively more pronounced in intensity and duration to the point it was always in the background by the time we flew home from vacation two days later.

Much of the remainder of this book will be about my recent Mental Illness crisis, decals of tragedy and pain for sure, but also some of triumph. One decal that will stick for sure is one of two Mental Health units I was in twice between Christmas time of 2016 and the end of March/early April 2017. My image then, although more positively altered now, is that a person does not go into a lockdown mental health unit unless things are really bad. I now have entered that semi-exclusive club that is whispered about. The following poem is an introduction; with hospital wrist badge for scanning, one drum beat of the unit was getting meds and having vitals checks with the introductory question from staff – name and birthdate.

Name and Birthdate

Inpatient Mental Health
Mind void of wealth
Adds to humiliate
What's your name and birthdate

Shoelaces and belt
To lockup they go
Assigned a roommate
Name and birthdate

Beginning – an empty stare
Is this real or fair?
Easy to deflate
Name and birthdate

Noise, bed checks
And locked bathroom too
My short term fate
Name and birthdate

Movies and yoga
Therapy and group
Not too late?
Name and birthdate

Calls and visits
Homemade goodies too
Mood does inflate
Name and birthdate

Pill cups and prescrips
Monitor for changes
Get it straight
Name and birthdate

MICK HUMBERT

Fifty-five lounge laps
Makes a mile
Normalcy impersonate
Name and birthdate

Real heavy chairs
Throwing a no-no
On mood do wait
Name and birthdate

Food Selection here
Less than other floors
Stabilized my weight
Name and birthdate

One drug - withdrawals
Another drug syncope too
Speak up to negotiate
Name and birthdate

Stable enough to
Discharge into world
Third time through gate
Name and birthdate

Out this time
To celebrate and liberate?
Absent now giving
Name and birthdate

Last Inpatient Mental Health Stay
Knowing of Discharge –Early April 2017

A Bit Sticky

Sticky - Assisted and Long-Term Care Senior Living is a tough business with thin margins based on occupancy. Keep the rooms fully occupied, OK; but if not, the red can start flowing.

Sticky - As the boomers start entering the senior living situations, more and more assisted living establishments are popping up. But this means that an ever-increasing number of front-line staff will be needed. The employment opportunities are there, but fewer seem to want this type of work; certainly not enough to keep pace.

Sticky - Nurses can earn more in other fields of work, so fully staffing those ranks is a challenge as well. While stable in some areas where I work, I have also seen a revolving door in key management and nursing positions.

Sticky - No great secret that the frontline Housekeeping, Resident Assistants, and Certified Nursing Assistants do not make that much money.

Sticky - With a declining workforce compared to need, and a tendency for higher staff turnover, the burden falls more and more on those who stay not for a number of years, but who are dedicated to their work. Burnout and a number of other less than favorable mental and emotional challenges are definitely in play.

Stickier still - All this when the price per month for nearly Independent Assisted living on one end to Long Term Care (aka previous Nursing Home image) is in the thousands of dollars.

Stickiest of all - From everything from quality of food to quality of life, from waiting to be toileted to waiting for personal affirmation, even with existing staff doing the very best they can, I ponder whether residents are getting sufficient "bang for their buck." As one resident in Assisted Living residence stated during a Resident Council meeting over the quality of the meals, "I pay thousands of dollars a month, and they will wheel me out of here on a gurney, wouldn't you think I could at least get a decent meal?"

Lamentations 1:12-13
Is it nothing to you, all you who pass by?
Look, and see if there is any sorrow like my sorrow,
which is brought on me,
with which Yahweh has afflicted me
in the day of his fierce anger.
From on high has he sent fire into my bones,
and it prevails against them.
He has spread a net for my feet.
He has turned me back.
He has made me desolate and I faint all day long.

Deflating

Tire pressure is something I pay attention to almost daily when I am riding. Even on a longer self-supported ride, I would check and correctly inflate the tires as often as I could. When at home or on a multi-week ride with support, I would inflate tires correctly every day. Too much pressure and you risk the increased possibility of a tube puncturing or bursting. Too little pressure and you increase the surface area of the tire contacting the road, thus slowing you down.

In describing Bipolar II (Agitative Depression) for myself anyway, both extremes are present at the same time. Anxiety and emotions run rampant to the point that you do not feel comfortable in your own skin; your brain is about to burst. During this most recent episode, and for the first time, it affected my stomach and appetite; I lost 15 pounds in a couple months. At the time, I didn't know better, but I was wondering and worried I had an ulcer from all the anxiety. I took over-the-counter remedies, while eliminating all junk food, dairy, and processed sugar from my diet to minimize any stomach irritation. At the same time, it feels like you are walking around with concrete shoes on; with the depressive side of the disorder it takes a great amount of effort to move from one activity to another. One description for the two I heard over and over in treatment is that with anxiety you feel a threat (fight or flight) and individuals get either very angry or want to avoid, while with depression you feel a total absence of engagement and want to hide.

Suicidal ideation becomes a battle; I have to say it was nearly intolerable. Even though I never formulated a plan, death was an enticing option; I can only say I understand from my experience, and empathize with families who have lost a loved one to suicide. There is nothing, in my opinion, that is cowardly about taking one's life; in fact, I consider those who suffer severely from major depression and anxiety disorders and live to talk about it - warriors and survivors.

If you are interested in disordered brain pressure numbers and when they go awry, look up statistics on the internet and you will discover similar numbers to the following for depression:

About 9 percent of American adults from all walks of life suffer from some form of depression at a given time.

At any given time, about 3 percent of adults have major depression, also known as major depressive disorder, a long-lasting and severe form of depression.

In fact, major depression is the leading cause of disability for Americans between the ages of 15 and 44, according to the CDC.

Many conditions may coexist with depression. Depression may increase the risk for another illness, and dealing with an illness may lead to depression. A common enough saying in mental health today is, "Depression is anger turned inward toward the self." It can therefore be very harmful to the body and self-destructive. In fact, according to the National Institute of Mental Health (NIMH), depression affects:

- More than 40 percent of those with post-traumatic stress disorder
- 25 percent of those who have cancer
- 27 percent of those with substance abuse problems
- 50 percent of those with Parkinson's disease

- 50 to 75 percent of those who have an eating disorder
- 33 percent of those who've had a heart attack

Depression is involved in more than two-thirds of the 30,000 suicides that occur in the United States every year. For every two homicides, there are three suicides.

Depression is also considered a worldwide epidemic, with 5 percent of the global population suffering from the condition, according to the World Health Organization.

Andy
It helps to name
Almost a person
My Agitative Depression
Taking away any fun

AN is for anxiety
D-depression in Andy
Y is for daily
Naming it comes in handy

Andy when present
My skin hardly standy
Life slipping away
Like fingers and sandy

Bottom of bottoms
Wish no one that grandy
Nothing holds spirits
Suicide seems dandy

Just out of inpatient treatment
Early April 2017

"Hello Andrea, how is the beginning of your day," I ask on my morning rounds as I see Andrea staring into the garden below; same place, same time, same demeanor every morning as I pass Andrea on the way to the Transitional Care Unit to do rounds. "Why am I still here? Why hasn't God taken me yet?" I get down to Andrea's wheelchair height, look her in the eyes, and simply say "I do not know." Andrea shakes her head. I ask if there is anything on the schedule of events that she will be doing today, like the singing group coming in after lunch. "No, I don't care much for that folksy music much. I enjoy classical music. I used to listen to it and go to performances with my husband often," she explains. With the ignorance of anyone who walks into a "foot in mouth" moment, I ask, "Do you have tapes in your room so you can continue listening to that type of music?" "Yes," Andrea says rather softly, "but in my room all alone I get sad because it reminds me of my dead husband. It is too hard for me." After a few more pleasantries, I give her a brief blessing. She thanks me for stopping by, then returns to gazing into the garden below with the stare that seems to be looking for something but nothing at the same time.

Andy cruises outside most any day he can in his scooter; his farmer tan gives bronze testament to his routine. Andy is younger than most in Assisted living, a terrible accident left him four wheeling instead of two. Testing the terrain a bit, I recognized that he liked friendly guy banter, like two elementary school age boys who slug each other just hard enough so each knew they were buddies. So we established a back and forth, commonly sarcastic, and mildly insulting exchange between us. He had become fond of a somewhat older female who was living there as well. They enjoyed each other's company; they proclaimed each other as boyfriend and girlfriend. Andrea was a person of sweet disposition, but not cognitively complex at all. Dementia started to set in for her and she needed to move to the early-stage memory care unit. A partial sadness came over Andy as he was not able to visit and see Andrea for the same length of time or in the same way as before. To add salt to an open emotional wound, Andrea met another fellow in the memory care unit and they soon became inseparable. Andy stated to me with sad reluctance, "That he was happy for her." The spark in bantering with Andy does not fit any longer, as most of the sparkle in his eyes has disappeared.

❧❧

Matthew 23: 1-4
Then Jesus spoke to the multitudes and to his disciples, saying, "The scribes and the Pharisees sit on Moses' seat. All things therefore whatever they tell you to observe, observe and do, but don't do their works; for they say, and don't do. For they bind heavy burdens that are grievous to be borne, and lay them on men's shoulders; but they themselves will not lift a finger to help them.

Weight, No Wait!

Weight of a bicycle is an issue, but blown way out of proportion in my opinion. Of course, there is logic in that statement that a cyclist has to pedal every ounce around so the lighter the bike, the less effort. Cyclists will spend an increasing amount of money to shave ounces off of frames, wheels, nuts and bolts of varying purpose, and even handlebar tape. I typically think to myself, why don't they save the hundreds or thousands and just lose a pound or two of their own body fat instead? For me, it begs the question: Perfection at what price?

As described briefly in the poem, a psychiatrist told me while in my last inpatient stay that people who are conscientious, perfectionists as one type, have the hardest time with anxiety and depression disorders. Perfectionists see it as unfair because they will do everything "right" and still can succumb to the illness. In my case and opinion, I live a much "cleaner" life than most. Some people could rightly reflect on their life and see how self-destructive it has been; they made "the bed they lie in." But not me, or so it seems to me. I don't drink, smoke, or use pain killing drugs as an out. I exercise and am not overweight. I take my prescription meds deliberately, and use light therapy in the winter.

So, for a recovering perfectionist like me, the "why me" question surfaces. I do everything right or what is asked of me to battle this disease, and I still can end up battling low grade episodes year in and year out, and even a major episode without much apparent warning.

Perhaps you know the type:

- A place for everything and everything in its place
- If not done right, it's not worth doing at all
- A job well done (not good or OK, but well)
- Going from room A to B for a particular purpose and seeing something a wee bit off on the way and it's distracting enough to correct at that very moment
- Check, double check, even triple check at times
- Little things bug you
- People with a laissez faire attitude bug you
- Simply typing initial drafts of a chapter of a book and going back to correct misspellings immediately as you see them

Don't get me wrong. High standards and expectations along with attention to detail have served me well; for instance, in doing dental surgery procedures. But when such perfectionism allows a person less time to, in a sense, breathe, the resulting anxiety may not be healthy. In my case, chronic back pain pokes and prods at me enough to increase anxiety and I have had to learn to train myself to know when enough is enough. Even though it is very logical, I am now only learning that certain habits and behaviors can do the same. I must learn to let some things go, to ease off on the brain strain just like I have learned to ease off on back strain.

Nightmare Conscientious

A statement stuck
A ...trist did share
That the conscientious
Not as well do fare

With Mental Illness
Those who wear
The perfectionist tend
to pull out hair

Do all things right
I do compare
So why still ill
Doesn't seem fair

If anxiety too high
Most difficult to bear
Hope drifts away
Virtual nightmare

Meds a necessity
When anxiety do stare
To calm oneself
Bring back some flair

Then depression remains
Apathy and despair
Trying to motivate
Like wrestling a bear

Ride the pony
Therapist did dare
Ease up on self
Bring back self-care

Shortly after last inpatient mental health discharge
Early April 2017

Psalm 119:105
Your word is a lamp to my feet,
and a light for my path.

Living on the Edge

Before adding a few adaptive parts to this bicycle built for the blues, it seems necessary for me to explain the terrain I presently travel daily with my Mental Illness. The analogy I will use is a busy two-lane road with only a gravel shoulder. It is tense riding with some carefree moments. There is the ever present and heightened anxiety traffic to the left with the very real risk of bumps or collisions. It dictates looking in the side mirror of life and being vigilant against the next potential risk coming up the road. Yes, I could just pull off into the gravel shoulder, but that could risk not only the possible flats of deep depression, but the mild form of depression for sure as it slows down the progress and joy of life. And so, I live on the edge, riding that thin white line of life while being scared of the depressive shoulder on the right and vigilant of the anxiety traffic to the left.

So in riding, as I will suggest in a life with Mental Illness, how does one have some semblance of a normal ride through life; not drifting too far left or right, while having time to lift one's head high and be grateful for the beauty that surrounds you. A strong hint is in the scripture passage from the Hebrew Scriptures above that alludes to God's presence. It will be enough to give light for your next step and also enough light to take that step in a given direction. Secular language would say, have an overall plan and then take it one day at a time. This has become increasingly true and apparent to me. If I take the long view,

I can best keep my life going in the chosen direction while avoiding the big potholes. But when I see, feel, or sense trouble coming, I pay close attention enough to avoid it if possible or brace for the impact if necessary. Sometimes, the disease will rear its ugly head, and holding on for the impact of depression and/or anxiety is necessary. But that does not mean that your focus becomes too acute, where your head is down all the time because you think all there is are bumps and potholes; this will cause you to drift dangerously into the traffic of anxiety or off the road into depression.

As a psychiatrist during my last inpatient Mental Health stay said to me, "You have to allow yourself to be sick." As a person that manages a chronic Mental Illness, there will be flair ups, small and large on occasion. The closest thing to a clever secret I heard in treatment is that you "have to ride the pony." I need to go with the movement of the illness, accept there will be ups and downs, which will allow for a more fluid and graceful ride. In the process group the theme of making a "friend" of sorts with your illness was brought up many times; the analogy of you driving the car but the illness will always be a passenger. The illness is a part of you, but you are the one in control. To be honest, the first time I heard anything close to "make a friend with your illness," I thought it bizarre at best. The last thing I thought a person with Mental Illness needed to do was actually go toward the illness, embrace the illness, own it as a piece of yourself; the way "you are wired" as I stated earlier. A therapist said, "if you think you are going to beat your illness, think again. Depression and anxiety have been around for a long time; if you try to beat them, you will lose every time."

Living on the edge now; enjoying some health but oh so leery of the illness, I can actually say going toward the disease IS the answer. It's not about beating the illness, getting rid of it, or returning to normal; it is about managing an illness I will have for the rest of my life. Some 30 years ago, and over a period of time, I accepted that truth as it related to my back. My current challenge is to do the same with my mental health. Bipolar II is my friend; Andy as I have called it. Don't have to like it one bit, nor should I, but Andy's coming along for the ride.

To Thine Own Self Be Blue

In more normal state
Can float with each hue
Dominant Bipolar 2
Generalized anxiety, then blue

Beaten down too often
What does one do
Assailed and terrorized
Mind altering goo

Medication alterations
The old and the new
Side effects up and down
Who's got a clue?

What's the right combo
Elixir or stew
Time feels like
Pharmacological zoo

Welcome talk therapy
Solo and group too
Emotions do process
Keep them in view

More months than a couple
Perhaps even a few
At peace with disease
By giving its due

With acceptance and practice
Skills forward on cue
Increasingly normal
More moments to chew

Yes thine, yes self
The disease's mildew
Accept, not liking
To thine own self be blue

Just beginning the Outpatient Day Treatment Program
Early April 2017

Cadence

Enough Drugs to make your Head Spin

Getting closer, but before adding various components, the ultimate goal for long distance riding is a steady and smooth output of energy for heart, muscles, and joints to handle the day-after-day grind in the wind, sun, and occasional storm. Cadence is the word used to describe the pedaling rate while pushing against the pedals; ideally you change your gears with the terrain to keep approximately the same rate of spinning along with a similar amount of effort put into pushing against the pedals. If you bicycle for enough years, each rider pretty much knows their best cadence and effort output against the pedals for maximum comfort and efficiency. For myself personally, I spin at a rate of about 70-85 revolutions per minute while touring. Spinning too slow against too high/hard of a gear feels great for a while but you will fatigue easily, grind to a crawl, and risk injuring your knee joints. Spin too fast against too low/easy of a gear and your muscles will feel the strain and ache from too high a degree of repetitive motion. In other words, the secret is to find and train in a pocket of spinning rate and effort against the pedals that minimizes the beating that the joints and muscles go through while having enough energy to make it to the end of each ride day.

This analogy fits for the antidepressant and antipsychotic drugs I have been on for about 30 years now. Especially during this most recent mental health crisis, I began to feel like a pharmacological guinea pig as my tried and true Paxil "pooped out" and the trial and error of finding another drug cocktail/magic elixir began. As a psychiatrist stated, other things such as exercise, diet, support, and light therapy would have as much bearing on my mental health. I believe that to be true, but I had those "in the bag" already, so the drugs became the main additional factor to get fine-tuned. As the poem will spell out, a few have worked out great while others not so much, and a few had side effects hard to tolerate.

I do believe medication is helpful, and a necessary assist in my treatment. It is also true in my case that the medications have side effects that need to be managed as well. Using the cadence analogy, the drug regimen makes the highs/anxiety not so high or out of control or the lows/depression not such a dark hole. My current drug regimen leaves me a bit fatigued and tired during the first 12 hours of the cycle. This is great for nighttime sleep when I take the anti-anxiety med, but it does stay with me a while into the work day, causing me to feel tired and sluggish. So, medications are necessary friends assisting in keeping yourself within an acceptable emotional spin rate for life, but foes as well. With Mental Illness treatment, one needs to not only manage the illness but also the medication side effects as well.

Friends or Foes

I wish to introduce
Acquaintances of mine
When they help out
Are indeed very fine

Depression and anxiety
Topic at hand
Some 30 years now
My body to land

Meet Axel, Traz, and Zack
Simba and Cyril too
2 Pams and 2 Bussys
All pills, some old – some new

Yuck to Zack
Over 25 years ago
Very first attempt
Mood altering amigo

Lost 8 pounds
Night sweats – 3 days
Abandoned immediately
Gotta be another way

Enter Axel
Friend 25 years
Relief did come from
Terror and the tears

Added first Bussy
Some 15 years back
Help out in winter
SAD did attack

On pleasant vacation
8th December '16
Knew instantly feeling
anxiety very mean

Had deserted Axel
That fall to test
Could Bussy be
My only constant guest?

Oh no, not again!
Quick get Axel!!
Panic to assuage
More than a little?

In just 3 weeks
High anxiety setback
Reached out to Doc
I'm out of whack

Suggested another Bussy
And add a Pam
Symptoms to cover
Was almost a sham

Overwhelming struggle
Safe in skin was not
First inpatient visit
Suicidal thoughts now got

Get off the Bussys
Up on Axel do wait
Add Traz for sleep
To welcome or hate

MICK HUMBERT

Got up first night
On Traz to pee
Collapse in bathroom
Never before for me

Home number of weeks
Axel to tweak
Anxiety still present
Not hopeful but bleak

2nd inpatient visit
Close to bottom did fall
Suicidal thoughts and nausea
Much weight loss did call

Some brief hope
Different Pam did find
Tapering off Axel
Cimba for my mind

Short stay at home
Hard to discern
Taper off Axel
Another crisis did burn

4 short months
Now 3rd inpatient visit
Broken and beaten
Screaming, I've had it!!

Cimba does continue
Axel still taper
Enter Syril for me
Looks good on paper

Traz and Syril
Together at night
Collapse to floor
Family given a fright

Epilepsy unit
Wired up galore
Cat scan make sure
Eliminate why floor

All clear was given
Bottom of bottoms did hit
Just bad syncope
Really, no sh_ _

Syril makes dizzy
Was told by .....trist
Eliminate Traz myself
Clear mood – no mist

Got off Axel
Decreasing limb zaps
Akin to finger in socket
But lighter if map

Discharge to home
Cimba and Syril only
Better each day
Feeling less lonely

Tentative now, but
Less second guessing
Truly on my way
Renewed hope – a blessing?

MICK HUMBERT

While glad for meds
But they can "poop out"
Hell to switch over
Mind wants to shout

So meet my friends
And also my foes
Poop out and side effects
Down to my toes

In chronological order
You may have guessed
The following drugs
My body as guest

Zack is Prosac
And Axel is Paxil
Added bupropion for SAD
Life rotated – my axle

In the first panic
Buspar Dr's fad
With alprazolam for anxiety
Known Xanax did add

In first lock-up
Trazadone now too
Better sleep for sure
erratic BP new

2nd crisis decide
Paxil must go
Add lorazepam for anxiety
Improvement did show

This time a charm?
Cymbalta - Seroquel gig
Near normalcy now
Pharmo guinea pig.

New diagnosis
Bipolar two
Prayer for success
to anxiety - blues

First week of the Day Treatment Program
Early April 2017

2 Timothy 4:6-8
For I am already being offered, and the time of my departure has come.
I have fought the good fight. I have finished the course. I have kept the
faith. From now on, the crown of righteousness is stored up for me,
which the Lord, the righteous judge, will give to me on that day; and
not to me only, but also to all those who have loved his appearing.

The Finish Line?

Finally, before adding a few adaptive components to my bicycle built for the blues, I wish to comment on the joy and oddity of seemingly coming out of the acute nature of a mental health crisis, when things seem to return to "normal." In a similar way to the scripture verses above, it does feel like I was departing from something as my emotions and thoughts settled. It certainly was a fight, if not a war, within my mind. Yes, I finished a brutal course and reawakened to the reality of living with a Mental Illness. I wouldn't go as far as saying it is a crowning achievement, but yes, faith in myself and a future was kept because I did not succumb to my suicidal thoughts. To finish the scripture analogy then, has there been a judgment I can state now, in hindsight, after the four months of hell I went through? What's the prize that I am willing to give myself, now seemingly out the other side of a major depressive episode for the second time on the cusp of turning 60 years of age? As I watch a beautiful yellow finch splashing in a pool of water at this writing, is it rewarding to say, "At least I did not kill myself or I'm still here?" Should I award myself for escaping by a whisker ECT (Electroconvulsive therapy) because the new drug therapy finally started making a difference?

It is shocking (ok, in good humor - every pun intended) to feel that I was an empty shell for one third of a year. It is shocking to know that I said out loud to close family members that I wanted to be dead. It is shockingly desperate to know that a bottom can be reached where I would entertain most any option in order to escape the mental pain: ECT, drugs, potential epileptic diagnosis, and yes, suicide. It does not feel like a triumph, a race finished well, or faith kept, worthy of a blue ribbon. That would be true if Mental Illness is something I could have avoided, or at least permanently beaten if I was strong enough, wise enough, or faithful enough. But as I stated earlier in the book, there was/is no beating this illness since it is a part of who I am. Just like a person suffering from cancer, MS, Alzheimer's, or any number of other illnesses, it is the "cards I was dealt." To no or very little fault of my own, it is how my brain is wired. So, to settle on a judgment, and find triumph in having survived another mental health crisis, the unwelcome truth that I have to accept is that there is no finish line. There never will be a finish line; ok, maybe, when I die, hopefully of natural causes, later in life. The race will always continue, pedaling with ANDY as my ride mate all day, every day. At best and hopefully for prolonged periods of time, the pedaling against depression and anxiety can be made comfortable by my approach to this journey with Mental Illness. But whether mild or strong, the winds of depression and anxiety will be a factor in each and every day of my life; always was whether I admitted it then or not, and always will be.

At least for me, after many sighs of relief - moments, days, or weeks now that the crisis is over, there is an oddity of reflection on what it meant, the decals that will stick, and what is worthwhile going forward. Any trauma I assume can be life altering, life threatening, life affirming, or linger post-traumatically. While I do not have a choice with the disease, just like my chronic back injury, the road I decide to travel with mental health is mine to choose. That was absolutely not clear in the midst of the crisis. I am not saying that the choice is easy or readily apparent, but what is worthwhile, and how to manage the illness, becomes THE question going forward. It has been no different with chronic back pain and disability, nor should I be surprised that the same questions are valid with Mental Illness. What type and how much job type work do I do? How do I back off and relax/heal when warning signs arise? Is it OK to be sick with the illness? How much and in what way do I involve my support system of family and friends? Is it OK to accept that it is not my fault?

Worthwhile

At Day treatment
2nd week do file
From bottom 3 weeks
Death's wish awhile

Stomach to normal
Absent churning bile
No death filled thoughts
My very essence defile

Now what!
Which channel to dial
Life's purpose discern
What is worthwhile?

Agony and suffering
4 months did pile
Now feeling better
How to reconcile?

When wife and kids
Clouded by the vile
How far can fall
Living life without style

Will learned lessons
Make more agile?
At bottom – a bit distant
Now a memory – a mere mile?

So, I pose the question
Over thinking all while
To what give attention
What is worthwhile?

End of 2nd week Day Treatment Program
Middle of April 2017

1 Corinthians 13: 11-13
When I was a child, I spoke as a child, I felt as a child, I thought as a child. Now that I have become a man, I have put away childish things. For now we see in a mirror, dimly, but then face to face. Now I know in part, but then I will know fully, even as I was also fully known. But now faith, hope, and love remain—these three. The greatest of these is love.

Mirrors

Vision and seeing things clearly, both what is in front of you as well as what is behind you, is of paramount importance in safe bicycling. There are potholes and crap on the road as well as uneven surfaces to contend with. There are few motorists, of all types, with crappy attitudes to contend with as well. The vast majority of the time, whether road or roadsters, there is no problem. But bicycling is a dangerous endeavor; gravel to the right, multi-ton vehicles going 60 mph three to five feet to the left, and any number of quirky imperfections in or on the road surface. The fewer distractions the better; no gawking at motorists, no earbuds in the ears, keeping eyes ahead and also looking behind in the mirror. Sure, there are frequent moments to take in the beauty around you, but vigilance is nearly constant. Any bike ride is cautiously relaxing.

I see my life's journey differently now; of course, any experience, especially hotly-charged emotional ones, will affect one's perspective. If cautiously relaxing describes the state of vigilance in bicycling, I used cautiously optimistic to describe my outlook when I was out of, or in the process of coming out of, the mental health crisis. It is like the sure feeling of taking the next step in faint light when getting up from bed at night and making it to the bathroom only by the dim glow of the nightlight. I felt normalcy returning for longer periods of time, but also lived with the searing recent memories of sky-high anxiety and the deep hole of depression. You no longer wake up with anxiety right there. Eating becomes a pleasure as the stomach settles, instead of a forced caloric intake to prevent losing more weight. You laugh more, care more, and see more to look forward to. Your vision starts to project into the future, instead of examining and fearing every conceivable pothole and challenge your mind can see or make up. If hindsight is a beautiful thing, any vision beyond extreme anxiety and depression is a treasure.

Normal

Out inpatient four weeks
Happy things not as dire
Medication in a groove
Albeit more easily tire

Caution is prudent?
Strong memory as crier
Need not look long
Brain in the fryer

Perfectly fine
Would make me a liar
But giddy as hell
No longer in quagmire

Saying goes - normal
Just setting on dryer
Still want to depend
Something wire to wire

Is it safe - all in
New normal - a buyer?
Day in day out
Each day a bit higher?

One month out of last Inpatient Treatment
End of April 2017

❧

Romans 12:2
Don't be conformed to this world, but be transformed by
the renewing of your mind, so that you may prove what
is the good, well-pleasing, and perfect will of God.

Pedals

In the chapter on cadence, I described how medications are used to assist the brain in staying at a comfortable spin rate; not too fast (anxiety) and not too slow (depression). In bicycling whether the cadence is fast, slow, or even coasting, the pressure all goes through the pedals. Whether regular bike pedals with or without straps, or fancy clipless pedals, some the diameter of a pencil and looking like an egg beater, all the energy in other parts of the body, especially the legs, end up being transferred to the pedals. Pedals are what make the wheels go around. When I go for a ride, it does not take me long to know whether it is a good day on the bike or whether I am having an off day. Pedaling tells me so; higher energy day and let's go for it, or slow down because it is going to be a tough ride.

Pedals are the brain in this analogy. With enough energy behind it, the wheels (soul) keep going round and round. That energy, that push, that force of creation that keeps a person in motion is the brain. If your pedaling is erratic, not suited for the terrain, does not supply enough or too much energy for the situation at hand, a break down in your life's journey may occur. In Mental Illness terms, the two I understand from my life's journey are anxiety and depression.

Anxiety would be pedaling with too much force all the time to the point of habituation and distortion of reality. Even when such effort is not called for, such as some huge hill to climb in life, the habit of anxiety can cause you to believe that more and more things are hills, if not mountains to climb. The common saying, "making a mountain out of a molehill" fits here. Even when there is no need for stress, or so much effort, everything seems like a big deal and the mind just spins and spins. The result beyond distortion of reality is fatigue and burnout. You wake up and it's there, spin spin spin, then crash from the fatigue and wake up again to the dizzying cycle all over again.

The other extreme, depression, is feeling like why bother to pedal at all. Flat terrains in life even make you want to crawl to a halt. Everything seems like it takes too much effort. First the temptation is to coast, but life must go on, and life does require some effort. You want to hide, you want to sleep, you want to totally disengage. To use the molehill analogy, all you see are mountains, even though they are molehills. Eventually, coasting does not work; you can't keep your balance when you slow to a standstill and you fall over. The brain wants no part of the effort, and the wheels stop going round; you give up and suicidal ideation results. In not wanting to move forward any longer, the will of the brain does not want to pedal and the wheels of the soul stop completely; let's get off the bicycle of life entirely.

With the bipolar II condition I manage now, just like in bicycling, it is apparent to me most of the time when I will have an off day. Two coping mechanisms or realizations I have found come into play having experienced this recent mental health crisis. One is that it is OK to have an off day, in fact, it is inevitable that I will have off days. It is beyond OK to slow down and pedal through that day or two at a pace that is manageable. The other is to trust to the core that an off day or two is not a crisis; the anxious or depressed feelings or thoughts are just that, and they will come and go and change with time. As with bicycling training and mindfulness, experience has told me how hard I can pedal on any given ride, it does not surprise me any longer that I should be just as mindful concerning my brain as well.

Off Day

Learning Bipolar 2
Condition to stay
Self must empathize
Too often off day

When smiles are tough
Much less be gay
To coping skills
Come what may

Temptation feels real
All day to lay
Oh, the conflicted mind
Tormented melee

The disease in part
tend to say
Runaway emotions
Having their way!!

So rise to occasion
Keep symptoms at bay
Maybe looking back
On par was okay

Recognize emotion
Behavior say nay
Disease as passenger
Not driver today

Accept the truth
Disease never slay
Some calm in the storm
Okay – an off day

Beginning of May 2017

2 Timothy 4:7
I have fought the good fight. I have finished
the course. I have kept the faith.

Shoo-es

If the pedal is your brain, your shoes are your mental attitude. I mentioned earlier that bicycling is a dangerous sport. A cyclist can get themselves in trouble by not paying attention. There are also a myriad of obstacles you have no control over. While weather and road conditions are the most obvious, the most unpredictable are motorists of all kinds. In my previous description, I used cautiously relaxed to describe this attitude, but that is when already rolling and into the ride. First the attitude in cycling that must be present is one of comfort, confidence, and courage; let's lace 'em up and do it. With any intense physical activity, it is all too easy for me to talk myself out of it: don't feel up to it, too windy, too hot and humid, or I'm too tired. But my own experience from riding has given me the comfort and confidence, courage if you will, knowing the feeling after having laced up the shoes and hitting the road is a mixture of peace and accomplishment that few other activities have given me. When successful at going for a ride, I shoo the excuses away and lace 'em up and let the pedals spin.

In the therapy programs I recently went through to assist me in coping with my Mental Health, one phrase that describes facing anxiety and depression is opposite of emotion. While anxiety makes you feel and think that there is a threat and you should avoid it, opposite of emotion tells you to go towards it. When depression feels like you should shut down and hide, get out there and stay engaged with life.

For me, during this last Mental Health crisis, my two biggest hurdles I had to overcome were the urge to just sleep (depression) and the urge to not exercise because I was too worn out (anxiety). It may seem over the top, but in all honesty, it took courage to not sleep too much and go for short walks. There is an overwhelming urge to run with your feelings, thoughts, and emotions and not even face the day. Opposite of emotion tells you to reconnect with the rational side of your thinking, leading you, indeed forcing you, to shoo your emotions aside, and to do exactly what you feel you should not. That takes comfort with the thought, confidence in your past, and courage in the moment.

C-Andy-Land

The topic of choice this
Poem now at hand
Is C as in comfort, confidence, and courage
In facing Andy-land

Anxiety and Depression
Daily is the brand
The hype, darkness
When life turns bland

When life is a struggle
Self-generated quicksand
Need comfort in fear
To make a stand

Opposite emotion
Courage is handy
Practice when difficult
Hold onto life's candy

When in mental distress
Takes confidence to act grand
Practice, pretend if must
Good habits on demand

Beginning of May 2017

Matthew 10:13-15
If the household is worthy, let your peace come on it, but if it isn't
worthy, let your peace return to you. Whoever doesn't receive you or
hear your words, as you go out of that house or that city, shake the dust
off your feet. Most certainly I tell you, it will be more tolerable for the
land of Sodom and Gomorrah in the day of judgment than for that city.

Seat

B4B - before back. Before I woke up one December morning about 30 years ago and could not turn side to side without pain, I was an upright bicyclist and a tournament tennis player along with being a dad and dentist. I had done no multi-day touring but had done long organized single-day rides around the Twin Cities. Bicycling on country roads had gotten into my blood enough that I had a custom touring bike made with all the bells and whistles on it. I had a full set of pannier bags and had done a couple two-day rides into Wisconsin to the family cabin. For about five years, as I struggled with back pain with no apparent answers for it, I assumed my serious biking days were over. With thoracic disc damage, leaning over an upright bicycle with some force transferred through the hands and shoulders to my back while supporting my upper body was a recipe for even more pain. And oh, of course even those high tech "banana" seats are still a pain in the ass, literally.

When I entered into serious rehab training with a professional for my back at a local exercise gym, part of the warm up for training was always to ride a stationary recumbent bicycle. Mmm - no back pain. I was the starting point organizer through my parish for a Habitat for Humanity 500 bike ride that was coming through town and I saw a few recumbents taking off in real time. Mmmm - they make road recumbents too. That winter, after researching recumbents, I bought my first recumbent, a long wheelbase Ryan recumbent with under the seat steering. 20+ years ago there were only a handful of manufacturers, not the dozens available today. I chose the Ryan because of its all mesh upper back support which, through the back strap supports, could be adjusted to fit. Starting that next spring, I started riding 10-15 mile rides just to get some exercise since walking long distances caused my back to ache, which also ruled out two other sports I enjoyed, tennis and golf.

The rest is history, as the saying goes. For whatever reason, when I am upright the force goes down through my spine and my back eventually aches. But when I lay back far enough, my back can take all the bouncing and pounding from cycling with no ill effects. Probably explains why, thank goodness, I have never had any trouble sleeping due to my back injury. Today, I still do some recumbent cycling in the winter at the gym, and probably average between 1000-2000 miles during the outdoor riding season. I am indeed thankful that there was an option B available for me to get some exercise while still managing my back problem.

As with my back injury, this second episode through a mental health crisis caused panic within me, to put it lightly. Option A with medication had worked for 20+ years and now it's Baaaack!! Rational thinking that there will be an option B, C, or D to try does not enter your mind easily when your mind is dysfunctional, out of whack, in a chemical imbalance. Besides, as I tried, and I did, going through various versions of drug combinations, the medications take 4-6 weeks to take full effect. When you feel the weight of anxiety and depression with suicidal ideation, 4-6 weeks waiting on a maybe, educated guess, a good hunch, is not reassuring. But my current elixir, potion, drug combo, after trying option B and C is now assisting my brain chemistry enough for me to say, thank God for Option D.

Option D

Saw yesterday
On TV, did see
Sandberg of Facebook
Lost husband, no we

She did write
In book - Option B
After life's adversity
Unbearable fee.

Sheryl did state
Resiliency as key
My daughter Teresa sees
The very same in me

Resiliency. REALLY?!
My ocean, my sea
Why me, this struggle
Now beyond option C

When option A
No longer can be
Author did state
Live the shit out of B

Really, all in again?
On at least option D
OK, come along ANDY
I bend more a knee

But don't forget
In bending a knee
I don't come anywhere close
To bowing to thee

Beginning of May 2017

John 6:68
Simon Peter answered him, "Lord, to whom would
we go? You have the words of eternal life.

Handlebars

In the chapter called mirrors, I acknowledged that as my health started to return it was possible to start looking into the future while being vigilant with my illness and not think every downturn was a huge pothole that would necessarily result in a never-ending series of difficulties. Better health allowed me to look ahead, and see the illness a bit in the rearview mirror. With this topic of handlebars, the obvious result in cycling of looking in your mirror occasionally for what's coming up from behind and predominantly looking in the distance for obstacles on or in the road, is that beyond seeing the obstacles you have to steer to avoid them. "Well, of course," you rightly would say, "who in their right mind would actually steer toward obstacles and hazards?"

But with Mental Illness, there lies the irony and trap. When in day treatment after my last inpatient visit, we talked about a concept visualized as a well-worn path in tall grass. It is such a well-worn path and the grass so tall that a person thinks or feels there is no other option. For myself personally, while I knew from my past that better health was possible, the crisis of anxiety and depression at the time made me think that there was nothing else possible; I would walk this rut seemingly forever with the tall grass of depression and anxiety to my left and right. In other words, I WAS my disorder, instead of a person who suffers from a mental health disorder that can be managed.

Even with medication, the reality of my bipolar II condition is that my brain is wired for depression and episodes of anxiety. The tall grass, if you will, will always be there no matter how hard I try to cut it down by fighting it. If I had a secret at present, it would be that while I need to accept that reality, I do not have to succumb to the depressive and anxiety rut that is all too familiar. I can steer myself, yes, with medication, but also with exercise, diet, light therapy, and above all, mindfulness, from that rut and cut a different path through this tall grass of my disorder. And no this new path does not mean using a machete to cut the depression and anxiety down; anxiety and depression are wise adversaries. If you try to beat them, they will win. The secret is to choose your own path amidst the disorder; in other words, it is hard daily work.

I used to think that becoming a medical professional was the hardest thing I would do. I used to think that bringing my A game to my work, day in and day out, was the hardest thing I would do. I used to think raising two kids so they could launch themselves successfully into adulthood was the hardest thing I would do. I use to think staying happily married now well into my third decade was the hardest thing I would do. Without equivocation, living with this disorder and trying to steer toward a healthier path while doing all the above-mentioned things is the hardest thing I will do. Put simply, I am still here and I am striving to thrive in spite of my Mental Health disorder.

Aim High in Steering

Aim high in steering
One answer driver's test
Good advice Mental Illness
From depression to divest

As on cycling road
Junk and holes are guest
High vision prepares
One to do their best

Perfect performance
Not goal, the quest
Overall worth and joy
Definitely do invest

Life bumps do occur
Need to digest
Real and attainable
Should self-suggest

More healthy thoughts
Even innocent gest
Helps rediscover
Most comfortable nest

Beginning of May 2017

Matthew 11:28-30
"Come to me, all you who labor and are heavily burdened, and
I will give you rest. Take my yoke upon you and learn from me,
for I am gentle and humble in heart; and you will find rest for
your souls. For my yoke is easy, and my burden is light."

Derailleur

There is a front and rear derailleur on most multi-gear bicycles; typically for three gears in front and up to as many as a 12-gear cluster in back. Besides the obvious of moving the bike chain from one gear to the other, the derailleur settings are important so the chain drops into, and stays, in a smooth-running gear. The frustration for a cyclist is typically when the front derailleur does not stay in a desired place and rubs on the chain or the internal or external stop settings are off and the chain actually jumps off the front chainwheel gears completely. The rear derailleur, in a similar way, can cause frustration when the settings are off and, with pedaling, the chain can jump from one back freewheel gear to another next to it. Put simply, a cyclist needs predictable shifting so they can concentrate on smooth pedaling and not wonder what small-to-moderate shifting annoyance is going on.

With getting better health back and over a long enough period of time, you finally get over the acute stage and panic that goes with it. Exactly what gear of health, and how predictably smooth, both started to enter my mind, especially with the side effects of the two new medications I was on; one an antidepressant of moderate dosage and one an antipsychotic medication for anxiety. I have noticed that the anxiety seems to be no problem, but being extremely drowsy and sluggish stays with me for a half day after the higher dose of the antipsychotic I take before bedtime. So since the beginning of April to this writing the end of June, I have increasingly wondered about the medication and whether it needs to be adjusted a bit for a more smooth quality of life. Don't get me wrong, if I had to choose between high anxiety with suicidal ideation to having some difficulty with sluggishness, I choose sluggishness. But I believe it is normal to want the right amount of medication and only enough needed to adequately assist my brain chemistry.

Just coming off a Mental Health crisis of four months, there is some trepidation over fiddling with the settings of my medication because of the real fear of returning to crisis mode. But with a psychiatrist's help, I feel that I can and should expect a better quality of life than being extremely sluggish for half of my waking hours. As usual, with these usual and necessary, but very potent medications, extremely slow and steady changes are prudent.

Is it Life or is it Memor-wreck

Tough to get settled
Coming back from disease
Anxiety and depression
New normal - please!

Is if new life
These drugs pharm tec?
Or still the same
Disease's memor-wreck

The new elixir
Or concoction so pure
Side effects some ways
Mimic "Andy," not demure

Am I unsettled
still anxiety
Or drug side effect
For sure plenty

Built in drowsy
Anti-AN for sure
Sorta like depression
Which has no cure

So "ride the pony"
As therapist did say
Life in general and
Disease & drugs have their way

Early May 2017

Psalm 145:18
Yahweh is near to all those who call on him,
to all who call on him in truth.

Cell Phone

A cell phone as a necessary part of a bicycle was unthinkable or unnecessary 20 years ago when I started to put on serious miles, and even days away from home. What seemed a "it's all on me" to figure out if something goes wrong has now evolved. As long as there is cell coverage, letting others know and then potentially bail me out when troubles arise when cycling is now normal. The typical troubles are flats and weather, of course, while having a solo or motorist involved accident tend to be the most serious incidents. With those who care for my well-being when I ride and know what I am up to, they rightly expect a call immediately from me when something goes wrong with a ride. It could be as innocent as, "I'll just be delayed getting home a bit" to "I am stuck under some bushes with straight line winds, lightning, and very heavy rain, and come get me" (a real incident that happened to me by the way). Depending on the incident, they answer my call and respond accordingly.

Mental Illness, in part, is a lonely ordeal; only you know what you are thinking and how you feel. Others can empathize, but no one truly can say "they know how you feel." True of any life experience, ultimately only you know. However, empathy and understanding by others can go a long way in settling part of your mind around the edges; the ordeal may be a lonely battle, but you don't have to go through it totally alone. Of immense assistance in hindsight were family and a few close friends who were willing to sit within and listen to the pain I went through. In particular, I honor most those who were willing to come visit me in the inpatient mental health units I was in over that 4-month period of time. I believe a common view in society would be, why would anyone want to go visit someone in the "nuthouse" or where a bunch of people are locked up for a while for being "crazy."

The poem speaks to one additional source of assistance; I needed to face my work situation as Director of Spiritual Care at a hospital and senior living facility. Between inpatient visits, I had already asked and received approval to reduce my hours, which has been very wise. Now after the last inpatient treatment, I discerned that what I was most passionate about was the chaplaincy portion of my job and not directorship. Both had a dose of anxiety in them with "the ask" centered around the unknown of what my two bosses would say or approve. Their answer could have been anywhere from accepting my mental health condition and recovery and approving my reduced hours and dropping directorship, to some other combination less appealing including losing my job entirely. In this instance, I was honored for who I was as a valued member of spiritual care given the work I had already done. They saw I had taken steps to improve my health (I was gone either at inpatient or in day treatment programs for seven weeks out of four months). They agreed I was more valuable to both organizations with the changes I requested, than starting over with someone else. To be valued for who I was as a person and not solely for what I did, was very affirming. Yes, when my health was at risk and I discerned a change was necessary, making the call and calling upon others for compassion and understanding was essential in moving forward with my recovery.

The Ask

To work re-enter
Management the task
To conclusion I come
To no longer bask

Agitative portion
Bipolar two
Management jungle
No relief, if few

With bosses cut quick
And make it fast
Tell of passion
Better sail on mast

No longer wise
Put on a mask
If don't want anxiety
To fill my flask

If they challenge/disagree
Don't feel aghast
Another human service
Will search to cast

Control of offer
Ignition, the gas
To future must point
Courage to ask

Early May 2017

Be sober and self-controlled. Be watchful. Your adversary, the devil, walks around like a roaring lion, seeking whom he may devour.

Flats

At some point, all the planning for a long ride comes to an end, and the actual ride begins. One way or another, it does not take long to find out why you prepare so long and well for a ride. My cross-country ride west to east started in a persistent mist. My south to north ride could not start at my anticipated site near Baton Rouge because of spring flooding. The first day of the Lake Superior ride I found out that I never thought of checking out the tightness of my pannier fastenings and had to jerry-rig a temporary fix until I could correct the problem through the gracious help of that night's overnight host. As recently as last summer on a five-day self-supported ride, I left early to get the ride in before bad weather was scheduled to move in around noon; wrong, as the weather moved in around 10:00. I needed to ditch into a local farmstead during heavy rain and lightning to get out of the weather under a woodshed.

The most typical reminder of a ride's fragility, unpredictability, and need to prepare are tire flats. On the cross-country trip, I had a flat on the first day out of the mountains in Montana. No big deal, I thought. I took out my spare and pumped it up with my bike pump. But alas, the brand new tube had a crack in the stem. Sorta no big deal, I thought. In the case of two flats, I always have patches with me that do a fair job of repairing a leak. After six patches and several attempts at getting going on my first tube, I was stuck with no other option. Long story short, I waited on the side of the road for 4 ½ hours for my ride support to show up again. Lesson learned. Now, I have two extra tubes with me on any multi-day ride, when large chunks of time will take place when I do not have another way out of being sidelined with flats.

Being two months removed from the end of the Mental Health crisis and feeling better with all my additional coping mechanisms, including medication, there are those occasional stretches of hours or a day that remind me of the need for vigilance and preparation. So here I will call them a flat period or day, when the air seems to go out of me. If you had never been through a mental health crisis, you would blow it off as just a bad day. But having gone through this twice now separated by over 20 years, you come to understand that life is good again not only because you have found patches that work, but that constant vigilance and preparation is prudent. Eat right at least the vast majority of the time, check. Exercise in moderation for sure several times a week, check. Get outside in the sun or use light therapy for at least a half hour a day, check. Take the medication as prescribed, check. Continue with nearly daily meditation and yoga (my most recent addition) to "soften" the mind to the stresses of daily living and chronic back pain, check. While a person with no health issues can bail on some or all of these and only have a bump or two in the road of daily living, I have learned I cannot afford such a delusion. I have a disease and it will never be cured. To keep the opposite, proper function and relative ease in living a reality, requires vigilance and preparation — check.

Dis-ease

Right on!!
The meaning to tease
Look at dictionary
Meaning to squeeze

"Apart" or "away"
For "dis" if you please
From all that affords one
Any type of "ease"

Emotions run wild
Bringing one to their knees
Sucking life's air out
A continuous wheeze

Not rational!!
Mind like swiss cheese
Holes poked - no hope
That depressive dis-ease

Second week of May 2017

꩜

Psalm 119:50
This is my comfort in my affliction,
for your word has revived me.

Riding in a Pack

When you are out and about in your car, especially on weekend mornings, you may run across a group of riders. Due to their common interest in cycling and relatively similar cycling skills, they arrange a meeting place, and plan a general route and length of ride. They ride close together so they can talk to one another, and as importantly, draft one another to make the ride easier. Many of them have logo-splattered spandex to look the part and to feel part of something larger than themselves. It is sort of a mutual admiration and aspiration club.

While I have ridden in packs on occasion during some of my fundraising group rides, I tend to ride recreationally alone by myself for a number of reasons. First, I ride a recumbent which does not pace well with upright bikes; I can do so on flats and certainly downhills, but an upright will beat me to the top of any hill because they can leverage more of their body in pushing against the pedals. Second, pack-riding requires much more of the attention be given to the closeness of the riding when drafting so as not to run into each other. Finally, I frankly prefer to be by myself, choosing my own pace while enjoying the scenery more.

As an analogy for my recent mental health crisis, being with others suffering in their own way with mental health while on my ride with Mental Health was an important part of the beginning phases of recovery. Whether as an inpatient or in an outpatient day program, the group, with the aid of a variety of specialists, learns each other's journey, listens to each other's current wild ride with anxiety and/or depression, and in some ways experiences the situation of others as well. As in a cycling pack, all the riders know and experience a similar ride while they are together. It would be an understatement to say that I was impacted by the scope and depth of other individual's experiences with their own behavioral disorder. Equally impressive was the ability of professionals to get meaningful therapy accomplished within a group so mentally dysfunctional. Finally, it is the gut and visceral will, soul if you will, of each person with a behavioral disorder that impressed me the most (more about this in the next chapter).

However, just like my tendency for bicycle riding, I gradually knew when it was time to go it alone. My Mental Health recovery was sufficient enough to wage the stormy and windswept issues of anxiety and depression by myself. In truth, I began to really prefer it that way. I would continue routine individual therapy, but the ride is now mine to make solo. Part of this feeling is that you want to get back to YOUR life. Another part of it is the feeling of fatigue and tiredness of putting energy into the group instead of yourself. And finally, like riding in a pack, after a while it gets taxing listening to and talking about other people's challenges - paying so close attention in group that you are helpful (drafting), but not bumping into each other (being insensitive). Group Mental Health sessions were necessary for me in recovery, but they do run their course. It rightly should be the goal of recovery to return to your own life journey and master your own route with a behavioral disorder.

Seas of Pain

When on the other side
At least a different lane
Group and programs
Make effort to train

Listening – do sit
Healing my self-disdain
Others mind in turmoil
Lit matches to propane

How to feel
Exit a bit more sane
Separation from group
Own health to sustain

Wish others well
No group as a cane
Leave group behind
Empathy for seas of pain

Second week of May 2017

Mark 2:1-5

When he entered again into Capernaum after some days, it was heard
that he was at home. Immediately many were gathered together,
so that there was no more room, not even around the door; and
he spoke the word to them. Four people came, carrying a paralytic
to him. When they could not come near to him for the crowd, they
removed the roof where he was. When they had broken it up, they
let down the mat that the paralytic was lying on. Jesus, seeing
their faith, said to the paralytic, "Son, your sins are forgiven you."

Drafting

If you are going to ride in a pack when cycling, the closer you get to
the back wheel of the cyclist in front of you, the better in order to
maximize the benefit of breaking wind resistance. As I mentioned in
the previous chapter, it requires constant vigilance to not only keep that
close a distance but also avoid running into the cyclist in front. Close but
not too close, as the saying goes. You quickly get a feel for the cadence
and rhythm of the cyclist in front; with occasional adjustments in your
own pedaling and gearing you can get "in sync" with the other cyclist.

The other assumption of drafting is that everyone in the pack takes
a turn at the front. No cyclist by themselves can keep the high pace
while indefinitely breaking the wind for everyone else. Cyclists take
their turn pulling out and riding to the front where the energy and
effort put in is increased dramatically for the period of time the cyclist
rides out front for the benefit of the other riders drafting behind. The
rider in front then waits for the next rider who feels energized enough
to pull in front and take their turn as well. This happens over and over

again, with varying durations of time depending on the strength of each rider in front. If speed is what you are after, drafting is the way to go; it is not unusual to increase a ride's speed by 3-4 mph over doing the same ride solo.

I was just finishing the day treatment program when I wrote the poem below; I wrote it to recite at my sendoff. A member who finishes the program is asked to share any thoughts, and the group members affirm the person before they leave the program. I remembered a lady in the partial inpatient program (all day but you get to sleep at home) I went through for three weeks in January after my first inpatient stay over Christmas of 2016. While we each wrote or said something to her in her sendoff, I affirmed her as a warrior. She had used this word to describe herself a few days before in group processing. Warrior would not be what most people would think of (I did not at first) given the description of her life; deeply depressed a number of times and going through more than one treatment program. Watching TV and playing video games was her norm; motivating herself to go grocery shopping or to do a load of laundry was a big deal. She basically described herself, but not in these words, as an overweight nonfunctioning hoarding depressed recluse. And yes, warrior is the word she used to describe herself. Those less sensitive and being critical from the outside looking in might say with apparent justification, "if she just got off her fat ass and got a job, things would get better."

This warrior desperately wanted to get better. Frustration and anger, as well as tears, came forth as she described her battle with Mental Illness. She was guilt-ridden and was fighting to not sink into feelings of shame. I do not know how others feel with other medical conditions such as heart attacks, cancer, diabetes, or chronic pain to name a few. People with medical conditions other than of the mind certainly can succumb to or add anxiety and/or depression while trying to cope with a chronic disease, but that is not their primary issue. So, I began to ponder the difficult situation that people facing a behavioral disorder have; how one has to try to battle through with the mind when the mind is the source of the disorder. How does a person think, reason, and feel their way through anxiety and/or depression when thinking, reasoning, and feelings have gone awry? How does a person think rationally when, due to a Mental Illness, they can't think their way out of a paper bag. How does a person feel normal when the mind tells you as truth that your skin crawls with anxiety? How can a person reason that there is no need to avoid or hide, when every fiber of your being tells you to do so? How can you feel no panic, no concern, no doom and gloom, when your diseased mind sees no way out?

In my view, it is not unusual for a warrior to be seen as a person who is willing to go to battle when the odds are stacked against them. Also typically, a warrior is viewed as one who stands alone in battle; this is where I separate from this normal macho image. I do think there are times in anyone's life when the odds are indeed heavily stacked against them; Mental Illness is one. Again, just look at a few suicide statistics easily retrieved from the internet. Two thirds of all suicides have a mental disorder as a key component. Every day 80 Americans take their own life (one every 18 minutes). 8.6% of people who have gone through a psychiatric/Mental Health unit will successfully commit suicide.

If looking at the glass as half full, having gone through three inpatient units in four months, two–day treatment programs, and being on medication for a Mental Illness disorder for 20+ years, I have a 9 out of 10 chance of making it through life without committing suicide. Sobering statistic. Warrior is indeed the word, but others must be at my side in battle to be victorious. Surely medication is a part, but other people both of the loving support type and from the sobering Mental Health community are as well. For sure, loving family and friends willing to stand by me during a crisis are irreplaceable. But those with Mental Illness who I listened to, learned from, and admired for the battle they are waging with their illness have also made my journey easier and more understandable. I drafted them for a while; they do battle every day, they are warriors.

The hidden treasure in the scripture above that few notice is in the phrase, "And Jesus seeing their faith said…" It was the faith of those that carried the paralytic, who made the effort to share in the paralytic's journey, that made Jesus say to the paralytic, "Son, your sins are forgiven." A warrior need not stand alone.

Warrior

Looking for a warrior
Most would not look here
Doesn't fit the archetype
those calm, no fear

But let's look here
At MI's interior
To those who aspire
motives superior

When mind goes
Into the fryer
Depression visits
Anxiety higher

Courage is not
Absence of fear
But acting anyway
In spite of it here

I say warrior
Here are the flyers
Looking at self
Health seeking buyers

So I exit the door
Time for adieu
Memories of warriors
More than a few
Second week of May 2017

Isaiah 41:10
Don't you be afraid, for I am with you.
Don't be dismayed, for I am your God.
I will strengthen you.
Yes, I will help you.
Yes, I will uphold you with the right hand of my righteousness.

Solo Riding

In the end of the poem that follows, I use a little play on words tribute to Star Wars. In one scene in Empire Strikes Back when Luke Skywalker meets Yoda in a hut in the swamp and says to Yoda about the Jedi training that he will "try," Yoda snaps back, "no try, do or do not, there is no try." In another exchange, Luke says "I'm not afraid." To which Yoda's voice deepens as he states, "You will be, you will be," with ominous music in the background. This duel between confidence and caution, between feeling healthy and still scarred, is how life is now after all the needed attention through the Mental Health crisis and day treatment programming afterward. It is solo ride time, out from under the treatment umbrella time, put your coping where your training is time, it is do or do not time. It is time to be OK alone, but not be lonely.

I have always been comfortable being alone with my thoughts and feelings, but there is a danger in becoming lonely and ill when things enter the anxiety and depression arenas. There is a purpose in talking through things and with others since, besides caring so much, they can give you pretty accurate feedback on how you are doing. The flip side of how I feel at times is that I am talked out, on analysis and feeling overloaded, and the situation has been sliced and diced enough for a while. But while appropriate in some ways, it betrays the reality that those close to me also went through their own version of coping and crisis in watching me go through four months of mental dysfunction.

With all that said, it is very true that no one else understands or will understand completely. A simple example, and there are plenty others, of this is that no matter how much women who are or have been pregnant explain it to me, I will never fully understand childbirth. Care, listen, empathize - yes, understand - no. So how do you explain being uncomfortable in your own skin? How do you give others a feel for having a mind that has lost control of a fair degree of rational thought? How do you adequately explain how it can take every ounce of effort and will to get out of bed, to eat, or to go on a short walk? You can't. The best I have come up with is to keep engaged with those who care for me, while not overly wearing my scars from Mental Illness on my sleeve or telling story after story of the mental decals that stick to this day. Living with and coping with a Mental Illness is largely a journey within yourself, by yourself, a ride done solo.

Solo

Oh the stereotypes
Pull up britches - pretty low
Or checked into the nuthouse?
Another thoughtless blow

I scream - no fairy tale!!
No gentle leaping doe
This is more a war
Mind screaming - WOE!

Hands plenty full
MI programs in tow
Working with others
More coping to show

Overall very good
Thoughts did hoe
When mind was less
Friend than foe

Applause is more in order
Mind mined & mowed
Coming through not broken
But certainly bowed

I soar again like the Falcon
Although coming slow
Put your hands together now
The adventure - hands solo

End of the second week of May 2017
Back to work

1 Corinthians 12:9
He has said to me, "My grace is sufficient for you, for my power is made perfect in weakness." Most gladly therefore I will rather glory in my weaknesses, that the power of Christ may rest on me.

Time to Ride

It is time. Time to continue the ride, the journey of life with a deeper appreciation of and a cautiously optimistic view of living with a Mental Illness. In Christian terms, as alluded to in the above scripture verse, is a feeling that the power of grace, of love, can be perfected in illness, the weakness of the disease. In being vigilant, and mindful, a more subtle approach to anxiety and depression can be attained, which allows for greater calm and purpose amidst the reality of living with an incurable illness. Whether by heredity, experiences including chronic pain, or both, the ANDY is coming along for the ride.

What I can say some 30 years into living with Mental Illness is, it is time to face honestly and objectively three truths. First, this bipolar II disease, while not my fault, will conquer me and make me falter if I think I can get rid of it or cure it. I can minimize its effects with prudence and practice, but it will be my daily companion. In those thirty years, the scars, the decals that stick from living with this illness, must also be honored for their effect on me. I can, and have at times, succumb to seeing my life as the illness, the sticky details and traumatic memories, but in truth I will always be more than this illness just as I am more than just chronic back pain. Finally, medications are necessary in my case, brain vitamins as I call them. But medications are not a cure or a reason to think the illness is over. Medications are one tool amidst others such as diet, exercise, talk therapy, mindfulness practice, and reordering your life around the realities of the illness. Just as with chronic back pain, which I had to swallow and then accept, there are a number of things I prudently should never do on a regular basis, so, too, I currently am swallowing the reality that I must allow Mental Illness to put certain acceptable limits on my life as well. Going forward, what I need to accept is that, while I do not have to like it, it is a ride in life still worth taking. The faith that comes from assent, trust, and hope that a vision of life with Mental Illness can still be, while different, filled with joy, be impactful, and grace filled.

Time to ride. Time to create more memories, indeed valuable and positive ones, even with the sticky decals of Mental Illness I have accumulated over the years. Time to stay connected with loved ones who see me as more than my illness, even when the illness can make me want to avoid or hide. Time to be of value, in leisure and work, to those around me that see that capacity within me even when my lowest moments with the illness causes my self-worth to take a hit. Time to accept and continue on with the love-hate relationship with the necessary medications, which assist in balancing out my brain chemistry even though they have undesired side effects. Time to be me, honest and open with the illness as appropriate, because this is, and will always be, a part of me. I cannot hide from it by hanging up this bicycle built for the blues in a dark closet; besides only reinforcing the disease in me, it would serve others who also have Mental Illness or love someone who suffers from it no good. To this end, mindful of my health, while grateful for any insight this writing has given to others, it is time for Mental Illness to ride more openly into the light of day with more understanding, empathy, and grace.

Head Space

There is a meditation site
So called headspace
Practice gradual and steady
Mind watching lace

Appropriate for ANDY
Anxiety - depression the case
When life feels like
Being squirted with mace

Desperately need now
Come face to face
More accepting mind
Loving self-embrace

Practice, practice, practice
Mind not about haste
The more engaged in
mindfulness - like paste

As saying goes
Mind terrible to waste
So prioritize mind
Meditating for grace

End of Second Week in May 2017

All systems - a go - again

Up and Running

Innocent comments
Others do make
When they see in you
What the illness does take

"Feeling better," they say
"Glad you're up and running"
As if the old self is
All that's worth gunning

Yes, brighter for sure
Life certainly more sunning
But to old self return?
When scarred life - no funning!

At least they are talking
Instead of merely shunning
But the illness is not merely
A one and done-ing

Well wishes by mail
Almost a fleet
Some who encourage me
This disease to beat

But that's the state
Of most less informed you meet
That it is just like a bug
That you repel with DEET

So running? Hardly!
Not from my seat
MANAGING is really
The essence and feat